UPDATE IN INTENSIVE CARE MEDICINE

Series Editor: Jean-Louis Vincent

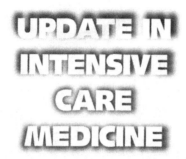

Springer

New York
Berlin
Heidelberg
Barcelona
Hong Kong
London
Milan
Paris
Tokyo

CORONARY CIRCULATION AND MYOCARDIAL ISCHEMIA

Volume Editors:

Michael R. Pinsky, MD, CM, FCCP, FCCM
Director of Research Division
of Critical Care Medicine
Professor of Anesthesiology
and Critical Care Medicine
University of Pittsburgh School
of Medicine
Pittsburgh, Pennsylvania, USA

Antonio Artigas, MD,PhD
Director of Critical Care Center
Sabadell Hospital
Associate Professor
Department of Cell Biology
and Physiology
Autonomous University
Barcelona, Spain

Jean-Francois Dhainaut, MD,PhD
Director of Medical Intensive Care Unit
Dean of Cochin Port-Royal Medical School
Vice-President of Paris University
Paris, France

Series Editor:

Jean-Louis Vincent, MD,PhD, FCCM, FCCP
Head, Department of Intensive Care
Erasme University Hospital
Brussels, Belgium

With 45 Figures and 5 Tables

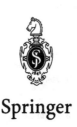

Springer

Michael R. Pinsky, MD, CM, FCCP, FCCM
Director of Research Division of Critical Care
    Medicine
Professor of Anesthesiology and Critical Care
    Medicine
University of Pittsburgh School of Medicine
Pittsburgh, Pennsylvania
USA

Antonio Artigas, MD, PHD
Director of Critical Care Center
Sabadell Hospital
Associate Professor
Department of Cell Biology and Physiology
Autonomous University
Barcelona
Spain

Jean-Francois Dhainaut, MD, PHD
Director of Medical Intensive Care Unit
Dean of Cochin Port-Royal Medical School
Vice-President of Paris University
Paris
France

Series Editor:
Jean-Louis Vincent, MD, PHD, FCCM, FCCP
Head, Department of Intensive Care
Erasme University Hospital
Brussels
Belgium

Library of Congress Cataloging-in-Publication Data applied for.

Printed on acid-free paper.

Production managed by PRO EDIT GmbH, Heidelberg, Germany.
Typeset by TBS, Sandhausen, Germany.
Printed and bound by Mercedes-Druck, Berlin, Germany.
Printed in Germany.

9 8 7 6 5 4 3 2 1

ISSN 0933-6788
ISBN 3-540-42037-1   SPIN 10797049

Springer-Verlag New York Berlin Heidelberg
A member of BertelsmannSpringer Science+Business Media GmbH

Preface

The coronary circulation is central to sustaining myocardial viability. Unlike the circulations of most other organs, if the coronary circulation becomes insufficient to sustain myocardial contractile function, overall quality of life rapidly declines and life can abruptly end. In partnership with the cerebral circulation, the coronary circulation plays a central role in sustaining life. However, unlike the cerebral circulation, whose function is self-sufficient to define life, the coronary circulation determines global blood flow and thus the initial state for the remainder of the body. This unique condition, together with the reality that coronary artery disease primarily affects people in their productive years of life, has allowed physicians and scientists who study the heart to enjoy a privileged position in the field of medical research and clinical practice.

Thus, it comes as little surprise that many new and exciting research developments involving the coronary circulation have recently come to the forefront of medical thinking. This reality, coupled with the large number of clinical trials of agents specifically designed to sustain or improve coronary flow in many disease states, makes the timing of this monograph relevant. The book features papers presented at a recent international symposium, the fourth in a series of meetings on Applied Physiology of the Peripheral Circulation. The papers selected by the editors review the most important advances in the fields of cardiology and the coronary circulation. Furthermore, the authors of these chapters represent the actual players in each field, the foot soldiers in physiology, captains of monitoring and generals of the multicenter clinical trials. This unique vertical integration of the coronary circulation from basic science through pathophysiology and, monitoring techniques to clinical trials is the fingerprint of this series and marks this volume as a valuable resource for anyone interested in the coronary circulation, from scientist to practicing clinician. This volume allows one to span this broad field in a condensed fashion but with clear high points.

The editors would like to thank the authors of each chapter for their excellent contributions and for the time they have devoted in their lives to making such contributions possible in the first place.

Michael R. Pinsky, MD

Contents

Section IV: Therapeutic and Clinical Applications

List of Contributors

X. Bosch
Servico de Cardiologia
Hospital Clinic
Barcelona
Spain

R. Cador
Cardiology Department
Cochin Hospital
Réne Descartes University
Paris
France

L. Capron
Service de Médecine Interne
L'Hôtel-Dieu
Paris
France

I. Carrió
Department of Nuclear Medicine
Hospital de La Santa Creu i Sant Pau
Barcelona
Spain

J.D. Chiche
Service de Réanimation Médicale
Centre Hospitalo-Universitaire
Cochin-Port Royal
Université Paris V
Paris
France

D. Collen
Center for Molecular and Vascular Biology
University of Leuven
Campus Gasthuisberg O&N
Leuven
Belgium

J.F. Dhainaut
Medical ICU
Cochin Port-Royal University Hospital
Université Paris V
Paris
France

A. Fernández Ortiz
Unidad de Hemodinámica y
Cardiologia Intervencionista
Hospital Universitario San Carlos
Madrid
Spain

J. Figueras
Coronary Care Unit
Hospital Vall d'Hebron
Barcelona
Spain

A. Flotats
Department of Nuclear Medicine
Hospital de La Santa Creu i Sant Pau
Barcelona
Spain

J. Gorcsan III
Medicine, Anesthesiology,
Critical Care Medicine
Echocardiography Laboratory
University of Pittsburgh
Pittsburgh, Pennsylvania
USA

J. Grégoire
Interventional Cardiology
Montreal Heart Institute
Montreal University
Montreal, Québec
Canada

D. Karila-Cohen
Service de Cardiologie
Hôpital Bichat
Paris
France

H.R. Lijnen
Center for Molecular and Vascular Biology
University of Leuven
Leuven
Belgium

N. Marin
Service de Réanimation Médicale
Centre Hospitalo-Universitaire
Cochin-Port Royal
Université Paris V
Paris
France

P. Sleight
Department of Cardiovascular Medicine
University of Oxford
John Radcliffe Hospital
Oxford
United Kingdom

C. Spaulding
Cardiology Department
Cochin Hospital
Réne Descartes University
Paris
France

J.-C. Tardif
Intravascular Ultrasound Laboratory
Montreal Heart Institute
Montreal, Québec
Canada

J.F. Toussaint
Service de Physiologie et Radioisotopes
Hôpital Broussais
Paris
France

D.M. Van Winkle
Department of Anesthesiology
Veterans Affairs Medical Center and
Oregon Health Sciences University
Portland, Oregon
USA

F.S. Villanueva
University of Pittsburgh
Pittsburgh, Pennsylvania
USA

S. Weber
Cardiology Department
Cochin Hospital
Réne Descartes University
Paris
France

B. Wyplosz
Service de Médecine Interne
L'Hôtel-Dieu
Paris
France

Section I:
Basic Physiology

Local Control of Coronary Blood Flow and Adenosine

F.S. Villanueva

Introduction

The control of myocardial blood flow is orchestrated by multiple regulatory processes, which result in close spatial and temporal coupling between myocardial oxygen supply and demand. The magnitude of coronary flow is a function of the driving pressure and the resistance of the vascular bed. Local control of coronary blood flow is mediated by alterations in vascular resistance in response to changes in the balance between myocardial oxygen supply and demand. In turn, coronary vascular resistance is adjusted by multiple interacting mechanisms including myocardial metabolism (metabolic control), endothelial control, autoregulation, myogenic control, extra-vascular compressive forces, and neural control. Coronary autoregulation and metabolic vasodilation are two basic forms of local coronary flow regulation. This review will discuss the local determinants of blood flow regulation to the myocardium, and will focus on the role of adenosine in this process.

Coupling Between Myocardial Oxygen Consumption and Coronary Blood Flow

In normal hearts, the oxygen supply from the coronary circulation precisely matches myocardial oxygen requirements over a wide range of cardiac activity, so that there is an equilibrium between energy usage and oxygen delivery [1]. Such a relationship is crucial because the heart is dependent almost entirely on oxidative metabolism for its energy. The resting oxygen content of coronary venous blood is low (25–30% coronary venous oxygen saturation), indicating that myocardial oxygen extraction is nearly maximal at rest [2]. Because of the high level of oxygen extraction even during basal conditions, there is little reserve capacity for increasing oxygen uptake when the demand increases. Significant increases in cardiac activity therefore cannot be met by enhanced oxygen extraction or anaerobic metabolism, so that increased myocardial metabolic requirements must be met by increases in coronary blood flow [2].

In the heart, blood flow appears to be controlled by the nervous system (neurogenic control), a myogenic mechanism, and chemical substances originating from myocytes (metabolic autoregulation) [3]. There is some evidence that decreased oxygen tension resulting from a decrease in coronary flow causes direct relaxation of vascular smooth muscle [4]. There are more data to suggest, however, that indirect regulatory processes predominate, whereby hypoxia leads to metabolic changes that result in the production of vasoactive substances, which then act on coronary vascular smooth muscle to cause vasodilatation [2]. These vasoactive substances thus increase in concentration only when coronary blood flow is insufficient, and decrease in concentration as the balance between myocardial energy demand and coronary flow is restored [5]. Metabolic regulation of coronary flow, therefore, maintains cardiac metabolic balance.

Several vasoactive substances have been thought to play a role in the metabolic maintenance of coronary blood flow, although the relative role of each has not been fully determined. Although the role of the nucleoside, adenosine, has not been fully elucidated, it has been hypothesized that adenosine is the principal metabolic regulator of coronary blood flow [6].

Adenosine as a Metabolic Regulator of Coronary Blood Flow: The "Adenosine Hypothesis"

The effect of adenosine on coronary resistance vessels was first recognized 60 years ago by Dury and Szent-Gyorgyi [7]. It has been posited that a metabolic regulator of coronary blood flow should meet the following four criteria [8]:
1. Exogenous administration of physiologic concentrations increases coronary blood flow.
2. Production by the heart parallels the increase in coronary blood flow.
3. Direct relationship between interstitial or coronary venous blood concentrations and changes in coronary flow (dose-response relationship).
4. Receptor antagonism or increased degradation blunts increases in coronary blood flow when the oxygen supply/demand ratio decreases.

Thus, for adenosine to qualify as such a metabolic regulator, it must exhibit the following characteristics: (a) Exogenous administration of physiologic concentrations of adenosine should increase coronary blood flow; (b) Adenosine should be produced by the heart (myocytes, vascular smooth muscle, endothelial cells) in conjunction with an increases in coronary blood flow; (c) There should be a "dose-response" relationship between adenosine concentrations in the interstitial fluid or coronary venous blood and coronary blood flow changes; and (d) Adenosine antagonists (e.g. receptor antagonists such as the methylxanthines or inhibitors of synthesis such as 5'-nucleotidase inhibitors) or agents that increase adenosine degradation (e.g. adenosine deaminase) should blunt increases in coronary blood flow induced by a decrease in the relative oxygen supply/demand ratio. There is extensive experimental evidence demonstrating that many, although not all, of these criteria are met by adenosine.

The adenosine hypothesis proposes that adenosine is an endogenous dilator of coronary vessels that is released in the presence of reduced myocardial oxygen supply or increased myocardial demand [8]. It has been shown that adenosine is released from the heart during conditions associated with diminished oxygen supply relative to demand (ischemia, hypoxia, increased oxygen consumption) [9–11]. Conversely, when excess oxygen is supplied by overperfusion, adenosine release decreases [12]. Similar relationships between blood flow and adenosine release have been described in the brain [13].

Adenosine is an active vasodilator [8]. Intra-arterial adenosine injection in the isolated perfused heart causes marked coronary dilation at concentrations of 10^{-7}–10^{-6} M, and maximal dilation at 10^{-5} M (dose-response relationship; criterion 2) [12]. In the blood-perfused heart, adenosine causes marked coronary vasodilation at concentrations even lower than that reached during ischemia [14]. Canine coronary arteries pre-constricted with norepinephrine or KCl relax in the presence of adenosine (10^{-6} M) [15].

Role of Adenosine in Coronary Hyperemic Flow Due to Ischemia and Increased Myocardial Energy Demand: Evidence for the Adenosine Hypothesis

When myocardial oxygen demand increases during exercise or cardiac pacing, adenosine release increases, a finding that fulfills the second criterion for a metabolic regulator of flow [16]. Dose-response relationships between the amount of released endogenous adenosine and degree of increase in blood flow have been described in brain [13], skeletal muscle [17], and cardiac muscle [12] (criterion 3). It has been reported that levels of adenosine in epicardial fluid co-vary with changes in cardiac energy metabolism induced by norepinephrine in isolated perfused guinea pig hearts [18].

There is conflicting data, however, regarding the role of adenosine during exercise. For example, 8-phenyltheophylline does not alter exercise-induced coronary vasodilation [19]. Moreover, in the unstressed heart, adenosine deaminase has no effects on coronary resistance, and does not affect the degree of reactive hyperemia during exercise in conscious dogs [20]. Such data suggest that although adenosine may increase with exercise, it may not be obligatory for increasing coronary blood flow with exercise in normal hearts. More recently, Druckner et al. have reported that K_{ATP} channels play a synergistic role with adenosine in exercise-induced hyperemia, since K_{ATP} channel blockade decreases coronary blood flow with exercise [21].

Adenosine plays a major role in the reactive hyperemia after myocardial ischemia. Administration of the 5'-nucleotidease inhibitor a, β-methylene adenosine 5'-diphosphate, reduces the reactive hyperemic response after brief coronary occlusion in the isolated guinea pig heart, and is associated with a reduction in myocardial epicardial fluid levels of adenosine [22]. Dipyridamole increases reactive hyperemia in conscious dogs and anesthetized cats [23]. Theophylline reduces reactive hyperemia after transient ischemia in dogs by 25%, and adenosine deaminase similarly attenuates post-ischemic hyperemia by 27–36% (criterion 4) [24]. In perfused hearts subjected to hypoxia, there is a significant relationship between tissue levels of adenosine, rate of adenosine release into the perfusate, and coronary blood flow (criterion 3) [25]. Systemic administration of adenosine deaminase blunts the coronary hyperemia normally seen during systemic hypoxia [26].

Despite the data supporting the crucial role of adenosine in the local metabolic regulation of coronary blood flow, it is likely that it is not the sole vasoactive factor regulating coronary flow responses to changes in energy supply/demand balance. When coronary perfusion pressure decreases distal to a stenosis, adenosine has been reported to increase to maintain coronary blood flow, suggesting a role for adenosine in coronary autoregulation [12]. The administration of adenosine deaminase, however, did not change vascular resistance during graded coronary stenosis [27]. Adenosine deaminase administered distal to a severe coronary stenosis in swine failed to reduce myocardial blood flow, suggesting that adenosine does not maintain arteriolar vasodilation in the presence of a critical coronary stenosis [28]. It has been suggested that interstitial adenosine concentrations are too low to elicit vasodilation during coronary stenosis and that this concentration does not change during autoregulation [29]. These data suggest that other mechanisms may be involved in the metabolic control of coronary blood flow in addition to adenosine.

Most likely, various vasoactive factors participate in coordinated fashion to regulate coronary flow responses to changes in the energy supply/demand equilibrium. For example, the reactive hyperemia following release of a 10- to 20-s occlusion is attenuated by 30% each by adenosine and nitric oxide antagonists. The simultaneous administration of these inhibitors blocks reactive hyperemia by about 60% [30].

Adenosine Metabolism

The predominant source of adenosine is myocardial ATP [8]. Adenosine is formed in tissue by 2 major pathways (Fig. 1): dephosphorylation of AMP to adenosine and phosphate, and the hydrolysis of S-adenosylhomocysteine (SAH) to adenosine and homocysteine [31]. In the heart, predominant sites of adenosine formation are the cardiomyocytes and cardiac vascular endothelium [32]. During normoxia, a major source of adenosine is SAH [33].

An imbalance between oxygen demand and supply is the key stimulus for adenosine formation [3]. During ischemia or hypoxia, the major path of adenosine production is shifted to the 5'AMP pathway [34]. An increase in the hydrolysis of ATP or a decrease in ATP synthesis leads to an increase in AMP concentration. AMP is then dephosphorylated by the enzyme 5'nucleotidase to adenosine. It has been shown that the enzyme 5'nucleotidase increases in activity during hypoxia and ischemia. This enzyme is found both in the cytosol and at the cell membrane surface of cardiomyocytes, and adenosine can be formed intracellularly or extracellularly [35]. Adenine nucleotides derived from platelets, adrenergic nerves, and endothelial cells are possible extracellular sources of adenosine [36].

Inactivation of adenosine occurs via three pathways: (a) phosphorylation to AMP via adenosine kinase and re-incorporation into the ATP pool; (b) degradation by adenosine deaminase to inosine; or (c) washout into the circulation [3].

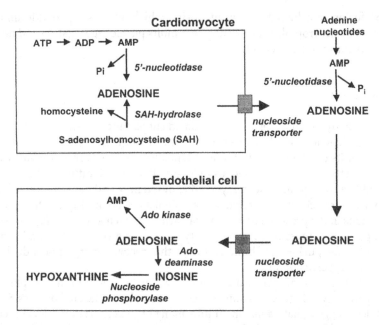

Fig. 1. Pathways of adenosine metabolism. The predominant source of adenosine is adenosine triphosphate (*ATP*). When oxygen supply/demand is imbalanced, the major path of adenosine production occurs via the 5'AMP pathway: ATP is hydrolyzed to adenosine monophosphate (*AMP*), which is dephosphorylated to adenosine. Adenosine can be formed intracellularly or extracellularly. See text for details. (Adapted from [3])

The major route of inactivation at physiologic concentrations is by phosphorylation to AMP, while deamination to inosine occurs at higher concentrations such as following exogenous administration [37]. These pathways exist in cardiomyocytes, endothelial cells, and erythrocytes. Adenosine kinase and adenosine deaminase are cytosolic enzymes, and adenosine is taken up by these cells via a nucleoside transport system which can be inhibited by nucleoside transport inhibitors [38].

Other Cardiac Actions of Adenosine

In addition to its effects on coronary flow via its vasodilator action, adenosine has a number of other protective cardiovascular effects that have been observed. The hemodynamic and metabolic effects of beta-adrenergic stimulation are attenuated by adenosine [39]. From the teleological standpoint, this may serve the function of reducing the energy requirements of the heart in the presence of decreased oxygen supply. Adenosine also decreases heart rate through inhibition of impulse generation at the sinus node and conduction in the AV-node [39]. Bradycardia during myocardial ischemia may be mediated by adenosine [40]. Oxygen radical-mediated injury by neutrophils, as occurs during post ischemic reperfusion, may be reduced by adenosine, which inhibits superoxide anion generation by neutrophils [41]. Adenosine inhibits platelet aggregation and may have an anti-thrombotic effect [42].

Conclusion

A large body of evidence has accumulated supporting a major role of adenosine as an endogenous modulator of the myocardial oxygen supply/demand ratio by virtue of its effect on vascular tone. Adenosine is released from the myocardium in the setting of a decreased oxygen supply/demand ratio, causing coronary vasodilatation, an increase in myocardial blood flow, and hence increased oxygen supply. More recent data suggest that adenosine has multiple other protective functions in the presence of myocardial ischemia, such as decreasing oxygen consumption by depressing cardiac activity, increasing glycolytic flux, and serving as substrate for purine metabolic pathways that recover energy pools during post ischemic reperfusion [3].

The regulation of myocardial blood flow during a broad range of physiologic and pathophysiologic conditions is a complex and multifaceted process. Substantial data suggest that adenosine fulfills many of the criteria for a local metabolic regulator of flow. However, despite the data supporting the adenosine hypothesis of coronary flow regulation, it is unlikely that it is the sole vasoactive factor in the metabolic control of coronary blood flow. Increasing our understanding of the relative roles of these factors in coronary flow regulation under different physiologic conditions will be important to developing a framework for devising therapeutic approaches to enhancing myocardial perfusion in ischemic coronary heart disease.

Acknowledgement. Presented in part at the Fourth Annual Symposium on Applied Physiology of the Peripheral Circulation: "Coronary Circulation and Myocardial Ischemia: An Affair of the Heart," Barcelona, Spain, October 1998

References

1. Boerth RC, Covell JW, Pool PE, Ross J Jr (1969) Increased myocardial oxygen consumption and contractile state associated with increased heart rate in dogs. Circ Res 24:725–734
2. Bache RJ, Dymek DJ (1981) Local and regional regulation of coronary vascular tone. Prog Cardiovasc Dis 24:191–212
3. Mubagwa K, Mullane K, Flameng W (1996) Role of adenosine in the heart and circulation 32:797–813
4. Gellai M, Norton JM, Detar R (1973) Evidence for direct control of coronary vascular tone by oxygen. Circ Res 32:279–89
5. Bruns RF (1990) Adenosine receptors – roles and pharmacology. Ann NY Acad Sci 603:211–26
6. Berne RM (1963) Cardiac nucleotides in hypoxia: possible role in regulation of coronary blood flow. Am J Physiol 204:317–322
7. Dury AN, Szent-Gyorgyi A (1929) The physiologic activity of adenine compounds with especial reference to their action upon the mammalian heart. J Physiol 68:213–237
8. Berne RM (1980) The role of adenosine in the regulation of coronary blood flow. Circ Res 47:807–813

9. Bardenheuer H, Schrader J (1986) Supply-to-demand ratio for oxygen determines formation of adenosine by the heart. Am J Physiol 250:H173–180

10. McKenzie JE, McCoy FP, Bockman EL (1980) Myocardial adenosine and coronary resistance during increased cardiac performance. Am J Physiol 239:H509–515

11. Watkinson WP, Foley DH, Rubio R, Berne RM (1979) Myocardial adenosine formation with increased cardiac performance in the dog. Am J Physiol 296:H13–21

12. Schrader J, Haddy FJ, Gerlach E (1977) Release of adenosine, inosine and hypoxanthine from the isolated guinea pig heart during hypoxia, flow-autoregulation and reactive hyperemia. Pfluger Arch 369:1–6

13. Berne RM, Rubio R, Curnish RR (1974) Release of adenosine from ischemic brain: Effect on cerebral resistance and incorporation into cerebral adenine nucleotides. Circ Res 35: 262–271

14. Rubio R, Berne RM, Katori M (1969) Release of adenosine in reactive hyperemia of the dog heart. Am J Physiol 216:56–62

15. Herlihy JT, Bockman EL, Berne RM, Rubio R (1976) Adenosine relaxation of isolated vascular smooth muscle. Am J Physiol 230:1239–1243

16. Fox AC, Reed GE, Glassman E, Kaltman AJ, Silk BB (1974) Release of adenosine from human hearts during angina induced by rapid atrial pacing. J Clin Invest 53:1447–1457

17. Berne RM, Winn HR, Knabb RM, Ely SW, Rubio R (1983) Blood flow regulation by adenosine in heart, brain and skeletal muscle. In: Berne RM, Rall TW, Rubio R (eds) Regulatory function of adenosine. Martinus Nijhoff Publishing, Boston, pp 293–317

18. Headrick JP, Matherne GP, Berne RM (1990) Metabolic correlates of adenosine formation in stimulated guinea pig heart. Jpn J Pharmacol 52 (suppl II):87

19. Bache RJ, Dai XZ, Schwartz J, Homans DC (1988) Role of adenosine in coronary vasodilation during exercise. Circ Res 62:846–853

20. Kroll K, Feigl EO (1985) Adenosine is unimportant in controlling coronary blood flow in unstressed dog hearts. Am J Physiol 249:H1176–1187

21. Druckner DJ, van Zon NS, Ishibashi Y, Bache RJ (1996) Role of K+ATP channels and adenosine in the regulation of coronary blood flow during exercise with normal and restricted coronary blood flow. J Clin Invest 97:996–1009

22. Imai S, Nakazawa M, Imai M, Jin H (1986) 5'nucleotidase inhibitors and the myocardial reactive hyperemia and adenosine content. In: Gerlach E, Becker FG (eds) Topics and perspectives in adenosine research. Springer-Verlag. Berlin/Heidelberg, pp 416–424

23. Berne RM, Rubio R (1979–1984) Coronary circulation. In: Berne RM, Sperelakis N, Geiger SR (eds) Handbook of physiology, Section 2: The cardiovascular system. American Physiologic Society. Bethesda, MD, pp 878–952

24. Giles RW, Wilcken DEL (1977) Reactive hyperemia in the dog heart: Interrelations between adenosine ATP and aminophylline and the effect of indomethacin. Cardiovasc Res 11:113–121

25. Rubio R, Wiedmeier VT, Berne RM (1974) Relationship between coronary flow and adenosine production and release. J Mol Cell Cardiol 6:561–566

26. Merrill GF, Downey F, Mones CE (1986) Adenosine deaminase attenuates canine coronary vasodilation during systemic hypoxia. Am J Physiol 250:H579–538

27. Dole WP, Yamada N, Bishop VS, Olsson RA (1985) Role of adenosine in coronary blood flow regulation after reductions in perfusion pressure. Circ Res 56:517–527

28. Gewirtz H, Brautigan DL, Olsson RA, Brown P, Most AS (1983) Circ Res 53:42–51

29. Hanley FL, Grattan MT, Stevens MB, Hoffman JIE (1986) Role of adenosine in coronary autoregulation. Am J Physiol 251:H558–566

30. Yamabe H, Okumura K, Ishizaka H, Tsuchiya T, Yasue H (1992) Role of endothelium-derived nitric oxide in myocardial reactive hyperemia. Am J Physiol 263:H8–14

31. Achterberg PW, de Tombe PP, Harmsen E, de Jon JW (1985) Myocardial S-adenosylhomocysteine hydrolase is important for adenosine production during normoxia. Biochim Biophys Acta 840:393–400

32. Belardinelli L (1993) Adenosine system in the heart. Drug Dev Res 28:263–267

33. Sparks HV Jr, Bardenheuer H (1986) Regulation of adenosine formation by the heart. Circ Res 58:193–201
34. Deussen A, Borst M, Schrader (1988) Formation of S-adenosylhomocysteine in the heart: I. An index of free intracellular adenosine. Circ Res 63:240–249
35. Pearson JD, Carleton JS, Gordon JL (1980) Metabolism of adenine nucleotides by ectoenzymes of vascular endothelial and smooth muscle cells in culture. Biochem J 190:421–429
36. Klabunde RE (1983) Dipyridamole inhibition of adenosine metabolism in human blood. Eur J Pharmacol 93:21–26
37. Van Belle H (1993) Nucleoside transport inhibition: a therapeutic approach to cardioprotection via adenosine? Cardiovasc Res 27:68–76
38. Isenberg G, Belardinelli L (1984) Ionic basis for the antagonism between adenosine and isoproterenol on isolated mammalian ventricular myocytes. Circ Res 55:309–325
39. Belardinelli L, Linden J, Berne RM (1989) The cardiac effects of adenosine. Prog Cardiovasc Dis 32:73–97
40. Shah PK, Nalos P, Peter T (1987) Atropine resistant post-infarct complete AV block: possible role of adenosine and improvement with aminophylline. Am Heart J 113:194–195
41. Cronstein BN, Kramer SB, Weissmann G, Hirschhorn R (1983) Adenosine: a physiologic modulator of superoxide anion generation by human neutrophils. J Exp Med 158: 1160–1177
42. Cusak NY, Houranin SMO (1981) 5'N-ethylcarboxamideoadenosine: A potent inhibitor of human platelet aggregation. Br J Pharm 72:443–447

Basic Mechanisms of Atherosclerosis:
From Inflammation to Infection

L. Capron and B. Wyplosz

Introduction

Myocardial infarction, the most common complication of atherosclerosis, remains a deadly disease. According to an international survey done between 1985 and 1990 [1], median 4-week mortality of acute coronary heart disease reaches the bewildering rate of 50%. Beyond treatment, prevention is clearly a major issue and any progress in our understanding of atherosclerosis can have a wide impact on public health. Inflammation is now ranking high among current explanations, with the possibility of infection as one of its potential causes.

From Possible to Plausible

In 1987 it was already possible, though somewhat provocative, to entitle a review article "Cause of atherosclerosis: the viral hypothesis" [2]. Data then available led to conclude that: "Intervention of a virus in atherosclerosis would help clarify the role of classical risk factors by accounting for some of their paradoxical influences. In addition, it would offer unexpected opportunities for prevention". More than 10 years after, the theme has matured up to being recognized among the innovative conceptions of atherosclerosis. Several steps forward have contributed: many studies, mainly bearing upon cytomegalovirus, have strengthened a potential implication of herpesviruses; bacteria, *Helicobacter pylori* and most of all *Chlamydia pneumoniae*, have added to the list of suspected microbes; and, at a more conceptual level, an infectious participation has fitted well with an integrated synthesis that views atherosclerosis as a chronic inflammation of the arterial wall.

Inflammation and Atherosclerosis

"The whole series of events that make up the well-known inflammatory process is therefore present": such were the words of Rudolf Virchow in 1862 to describe atherosclerosis [3]. His statement has since been amply confirmed. It is now well established that atherosclerotic lesions do display the 4 classical features of chronic inflammation [4]: (a) monolymphocytic infiltration – besides arterial smooth muscle cells, monocytes/macrophages and T-lymphocytes compose the main cellular populations of plaques [5]; (b) sclerosis – mentioned in the name of the disease, sclerosis usually comprises more than three quarters of the plaques volume; the remaining part consisting in atheroma (lipid core) [6]; (c) cellular proliferation – contrary to the healthy arterial wall where cellular turn-over is extremely slow, plaques have a substantial mitotic activity (1–2% cells in cycle) that involves smooth muscle cells, macrophages and lymphocytes [7]; (d) vascular proliferation – a normal endartery is devoid of vessels, but an atherosclerotic intima is richly irrigated by neovessels that develop in proportion to plaque growth [8].

Ranging all the way from the formation of plaques to their complications (stenosis, rupture, thrombosis), inflammation provides a unifying framework for the pathogenesis of atherosclerosis, that helps reconciling the 2 historical rivals: lipid or insudation theory, and thrombus or encrustation theory [9]. In essence, inflammation is the reaction of a living tissue against an aggression; its aim is repair; when aggression is repeated or sustained, inflammation becomes chronic and may overtake its aim, to become a source of damage. Beyond pathogenic preoccupation, viewing atherosclerosis as such leads to the fundamental question of etiology: which is the nature of the aggression or aggressions that ignite and fuel the atherosclerotic inflammation [4]? Established risk factors (e.g., cholesterol, diabetes, hypertension, smoking) are the traditional answers. Infection is a less orthodox one, but is neither new [10] nor unsubstantiated.

From Inflammation to Infection

Even if sometimes compared to an abscess, with its soft lipid core and its hard fibrotic shell, an atherosclerotic plaque does not look like a classical infectious lesion at fist sight. If infection plays any role, it is a low-grade one that implies microbes with certain discrete characteristics: a wide epidemiological distribution; a tropism for the arterial wall; and an aptitude for latency and recurrence that accounts for their hidden persistence in the plaque cells, with phases of activity that result in evolving flares, culminating in plaque rupture. Our attention should bear upon agents with such features, which disqualifies most common pyogenic bacteria.

Only the hypothesis where microbes are directly implicated in atherosclerosis because they infect the arterial intima will be considered here, leaving aside the alternative of an indirect participation along two possible models: (a) any infection, whatever its agent and localization, may trigger a generalized reaction releasing various inflammatory molecules in the systemic circulation (e.g., cytokines, fibrinogen, C-reactive protein, activated oxygen species, eicosanoids), that may activate the atherosclerotic focus in a non specific manner [11]; (b) an antigenic mimiory may generate an autoimmune response – an antibody raised against a microbial antigen can be cross-specific for a protein naturally expressed in the plaques, which would provoke an immune reaction able to enhance local inflammation; some bacterial heat shock proteins (HSPs) with a structure that has remained very close to human HSPs have been implicated in such a process [12].

A direct role for microbes in atherosclerosis can be deduced from several types of evidence. (a) Experimental studies induce in vivo lesions in whole animals, or in vitro changes in cellular models, bearing some resemblance with the human atherosclerotic process. (b) Using case-control or prospective cohort designs, epidemiology detects associations between occurrence of arterial diseases and serum titers of antibodies against the suspected infectious agent; a high prevalence of seropositivity in the reference population may however decrease the sensitivity of such epidemiological studies. (c) Several histology techniques can detect whole microbial bodies or, more commonly, specific microbial molecules (proteins, nucleic acids) inside human plaques. This may seem as a most suggestive demonstration, but the explanation of the "harmless hobo" should never be overlooked [13]: as any sites of chronic inflammation, plaques recruit and harbor circulating leukocytes, particularly monocytes which, during a former defense mission in an other site of the body (e.g., respiratory, digestive or urinary tracks), can have phagocyted and kept microbes in a more or less degraded state; detection of such agents in plaques then would not necessarily attest to their implication in the formation of the lesion, but would rather merely reflect its inflammatory nature.

A fourth and much more decisive line of evidence adds to the three preceding ones: to materialize all the potential interest of the infectious hypothesis by showing that an antiinfectious drug does protect against the clinical complications of atherosclerosis.

On such grounds, a viral family (herpesviruses) and two bacteria (*Chlamydia pneumoniæ* and *Helicobacter pylori*) have so far been incriminated in atherosclerosis. Their respective records of evidence for an implication, as summarized in Table 1, has recently been the subject of an excellent quantitative review [14].

Viruses and Atherosclerosis

Experiments with herpesviruses published 20 years ago [15] have provided the first elaborate clue to a potential participation of infection in atherosclerosis. It all began with the serendipitous observation in domestic cats that cultured urinary epithelial cells in become loaded with cholesterol when infected by a feline herpesvirus. Based upon this unexpected observation, chicken were infected with an

Table 1. Infectious hypothesis of atherosclerosis: summary records of evidence for agents that have been considered as potentially causal (+ generally in favor, ± partial or contradictory, – lacking or negative)

Type of evidence	Herpesvirus cytomegalovirus	*Chlamydia pneumoniae*	*Helicobacter pylori*
Animal models	+	±	–
Cellular models	+	±	–
Sero-epidemiology	+	+	±
Detection in plaques	+	+	–
Treatment	–	+	–

avian herpesvirus, Marek's disease virus. Arterial lesions with a striking resemblance to atherosclerosis resulted, displaying fibrous thickenings enclosing an atheroma. Since, many additional observations have been added, with experiments mainly bearing upon two human herpesviruses: type 1 herpesvirus simplex and cytomegalovirus. Although unable to provoke experimental lesions as striking as those recorded with Marek's disease virus, these two viruses infect arterial cells and alter their functions in a way that is considered as favorable to plaque formation: foamy transformation (cytoplasmic accumulation of lipid vacuoles) and proliferation of smooth muscle cells; dysfunction of endothelial cells with prothrombotic effect and expression of adhesion molecules; enhanced production of cytokines by monocytes/macrophages [16].

Most clinical data have dealt with cytomegalovirus (CMV or HHV5, fifth of the eight known human herpesviruses). In immunocompetent subjects infection is mostly silent or benign (mononucleosis-like illness) but the rate of seropositivity is very high (50–90% in adult populations), with a strong influence of social and economic conditions. Sixteen histology studies have used various methods to detect CMV in a total of 398 healthy arteries and 607 atherosclerotic arteries. The global rate of positivity has been only marginally higher in lesions than in control samples [47% versus 39%, giving an adjusted odds ratio of 1.4 with a 95% confidence interval (95% CI) 1.0–1.9]. Odds ratio increases to 2.5 (95% CI: 1.6–3.8) when only studies that have used more sensible genomic amplification techniques are taken into account [14]. The only firm conclusion to be drawn here is that CMV has a marked tropism for the arterial wall where its main targets are smooth muscle cells [17]. Eighteen epidemiological studies yield an odds ratio of about 2 for the association between atherosclerotic diseases and CMV seropositivity. Their small sizes and many methodological weaknesses mandate careful interpretation of this estimate [14].

CMV has also been implicated in two special forms of atherosclerosis: arterial graft disease, and postangioplasty restenosis. Occurrence of CMV infection, facilitated by immunosuppressive therapy, is often though not unanimously viewed as a risk factor for transplant coronary heart disease [18] Much experimental work favors the intervention of CMV in this form of chronic rejection, but histology data have been contradictory so far [19, 20]. For restenosis after coronary angioplasty, a study [21] has found a much higher incidence in 46 patients seropositive for CMV than in 29 seronegative patients: 43% versus 8%, i.e. an odds ratio of 9.0 (95% CI: 1.9–42.4), a value far greater than those reached by any risk factor studied so far. The same group has published experimental data suggesting that CMV interferes with the expression of the antioncogene protein p53 favoring unrepressed smooth muscle cell proliferation and restenosis [22]. A recent study tends to confirm an association between CMV seropositivity and coronary restenosis [23], but at least three others have failed to do so [24].

The strongest evidence in favor of CMV and, more generally, of herpesviruses is therefore experimental. Clinico-anatomical evidence is weak, and even contradictory. However, the weakness of histology data cannot overlook a remarkable feature of CMV: in vitro this virus, when infecting arterial smooth muscle cells, can durably impair their functions, but without leaving the least trace, even genetic, of its intervention (so-called "hit and run") [25].

Bacteria and Atherosclerosis

Chlamydia Pneumoniae

Formally identified in 1986 under the name of *Chlamydia* TWAR [26], *C. pneumoniae* is a gram-negative bacterium and obligatory intracellular parasite. It is a very common cause of respiratory infections: virtually all individuals are infected at some time in their life [27]. In 1988, starting from the observation that endocarditis or myocarditis can complicate *C. pneumoniae* infection, a Finnish team observed that high serum titers of antibodies against *C. pneumoniae* were more frequent in 40 victims of a recent acute coronary event (68%) and in 30 patients with severe angina (50%) than in 41 healthy controls (17%) [28] Seventeen sero-epidemiological studies published since have generally confirmed the association with an odds ratio of 2 or greater, but with the same methodological limits as mentioned for CMV, and the added drawback that serologic techniques have not always been very reliable [14]. Thirteen histology studies have been looking for chlamydial proteins, nucleic acids or elementary bodies in arterial tissues, with a positivity rate of 52% in 495 lesions, versus only 5% in 118 arterial samples without atherosclerosis, yielding an adjusted odds ratio of about 10 (95% CI: 5–22) [14]. So far, experimental work has failed to provide strong evidence that *C. pneumoniae* alone can induce atherosclerosis-like lesions in animals. Yet, infection can accelerate lesion development in models such as the hypercholesterolemic rabbit [29] or the apo E-knockout mouse [30]. Studies with cellular models in vitro are just beginning to come out [31, 32].

The strongest evidence in favor of *C. pneumoniae* has therefore been drawn from histopathology, but the "harmless hobo" caveat must also be considered seriously here [13], as the bacterium resides and persists mainly in plaque monocytes/macrophages (although some can be found in smooth muscle and endothelial cells) [33].

Helicobacter Pylori

The strong implication of *H. pylori* in peptic ulcer disease has been a major advance in gastroenterology, and has provided an exemplary demonstration that ignored infection can be the etiologic key to a disease traditionally considered as inflammatory, degenerative or cryptogenic. Since 1994 at least 20 sero-epidemiological studies have sought for an association between *H. pylori* infection and arterial diseases. Overviews have concluded to a weak and inconstent link of dubious significance [14, 34]. No experimental or pathologic data have been put forward to support such an association.

From Plausible to Probable

Such was the situation not so long ago: the greatest strength of the infectious hypothesis was its theoretical plausibility, in relation with the inflammatory explanation of atherosclerosis; many pieces of evidence had accumulated around CMV and *C. pneumoniae*, but none of them, when considered individually, had the power to establish conviction because data were fragmentary, subject to bias, or contradicted by other sources. A decisive impetus could only come from therapeutic evidence: no one has ever ventured to target CMV because available antiviral drugs are inconvenient (parenteral administration, high cost and toxicity); but the situation is quite different with *C. pneumoniae*, a bacterium sensitive to many orally active antibiotics that are readily available. In the summer of 1997, an important step forward has been the publication of two pilot trials using a macrolide antibiotic against coronary heart disease.

Gupta et al. (London, UK) [35] found that in 213 men who had survived a myocardial infarction cardiovascular prognosis at 18 months was correlated with the titer of serum antibodies against *C. pneumoniae*: it was four times better in seronegative than in strongly seropositive patients (titer ≥1/64). In these 80 latter patients, following partial randomization, treatment with azithromycin (500 mg per day for 3 days, in one or two courses, then separated by a 3-month interval) was compared with placebo. Antibiotic treatment reverted cardiovascular prognosis to the favorable level observed in seronegative patients. A multicenter trial in Argentina [36] enrolled 202 patients with non-Q wave acute coronary syndromes (90% unstable angina, 10% non-Q wave myocardial infarction) to test the efficacy of an other antichlamydial antibiotic. Following randomization and under double-blind conditions, 102 patients received oral roxithromycin (150 mg twice daily), and the remaining 100 were given a placebo. All patients did also receive conventional treatment against acute myocardial ischemia. Antibiotic treatment was considered as effective if taken for at least 3 days (with the objective to maintain it for 30 days). Primary endpoint was the cumulated incidence of Q-wave myocardial infarction, coronary death, or relapsing angina in the 30 days after the beginning of treatment. Per protocol analysis restricted to patients who completed the minimum 72-h active treatment ($n=93$ in each group) found 9 events in the placebo-group (5 cases of recurrent angina, 2 infarctions and 2 deaths) versus one only (one case of recurrent angina) in the roxithromycin group.

Although preliminary and bearing upon small numbers of cases, these results do lead the infectious hypothesis in the area of probability: the difference in favor of the treated group as compared to the placebo group was statistically significant (probability of the null hypothesis smaller than 0.05) in both the British study (chronic coronary heart disease, azithromycin, intention-to-treat analysis) and the Argentinean study (acute coronary heart disease, roxithromycin, per protocol analysis).

From Probable to Established

The two macrolide studies, although their methods and results remain open to criticism, have projected *C. pneumoniae* in the spotlight. Will it burn there like a straw fire or, on the contrary, play to the cardiologists the same scene as *H. pylori* has recently played to the gastro-enterologists? The British and Argentinean results must of course be replicated. More should be published soon from the

Argentinean trial (6-month results) and, hopefully, several large-scale macrolide trials are being launched. One of those, ACADEMIC, with azithromycin in postinfarction prevention, has even suffered slightly from the impatience of its promoters: although planned for a 2-year duration, its non-significant results at 6 months have already been presented (Muhlestein JB et al. 47th Annual Scientific Session of the American College of Cardiology, Atlanta, March 29-April 1, 1998). Hopefully, such an awkward breaking of the randomization rules should not occur again, and the medical community will serenely wait for the 2–4 years that are needed to reach a fair verdict on the usefulness of antibiotics to control coronary disease. Meanwhile pathologic and experimental results will rapidly accumulate, but without ever reaching the persuasiveness of positive therapeutic trials.

An embarrassing question cannot be put aside: has the chlamydial wave definitely drowned the viral track that nonetheless had lighted the slow match of infection in atherosclerosis? Probably yes, but 2 possibilities cannot be entirely ruled out: (a) atherosclerosis might be the univocal response of arterial intima to various aggressions by any of several infectious pathogens and non-infectious factors (e.g., metabolic, hemodynamic, immune, toxic), which would make it a multifactorial disease with multiple causes; (b) CMV and *C. pneumoniae* could be accomplices, the former acting early to prepare the ground (plaque formation) so that the latter, acting later, can express its virulence by leading to the thrombotic and obstructive complications of the plaque. In this regard, interesting avenues are open by modifications of smooth muscle cells transfected by CMV, such as immortalization [25] or foamy transformation [37]. Moreover, other pathogens may still emerge: herpesviruses have raised suspicion in 1978 [15], 8 years before the formal identification of *C. pneumoniae* [26]. A partial or even complete failure of macrolides in coronary disease would not definitively disqualify the idea of a microbial participation in atherosclerosis.

Conclusion

The best side of all this recent progress in the etiology of atherosclerosis is that the very idea of infection is now considered earnestly, and that the required energy and funds are now being devoted to testing it. We are still a long way from a "last nail in the coffin" debate. To be frank – between the atherosclerosis enigma and its microbial hypothesis – we are not sure yet of which corpse will eventually be loaded in the hearse.

References

1. Chambless L, Keil U, Dobson A, et al. (1997) Population versus clinical view of case fatality from acute coronary heart disease: Results from the WHO MONICA Project 1985–1990. Circulation 96:3849–3859
2. Capron L (1987) Cause de l'athérosclérose: l'hypothèse virale. Arch Mal Cœur 80 (suppl.I):51–55
3. Virchow R (1862) Phlogose und Thrombose im Gefässystem. In: Gesammelte Abhandlungen zur wissenschaftlichen Medizin. Max Hirsch, Berlin

4. Capron L (1993) Mécanismes inflammatoires de l'athérosclérose: inférences pathogéniques et étiologiques. Arch Mal Cœur 86 (suppl.I):19–30
5. Jonasson L, Holm J, Skalli O, Bondjers G, Hansson GK (1986) Regional accumulations of T cells, macrophages, and smooth muscle cells in the human atherosclerotic plaque. Arteriosclerosis 6:131–138
6. Kragel AH, Reddy SG, Wittes JT, Roberts WC (1989) Morphometric analysis of the composition of atherosclerotic plaques in the four major epicardial coronary arteries in acute myocardial infarction and in sudden coronary death. Circulation 80:1747–1756
7. Rekhter MD, Gordon D (1995) Active proliferation of different cell types, including lymphocytes, in human atherosclerotic plaques. Am J Pathol 147:668–677
8. Zhang Y, Cliff WJ, Schoefl GI, Higgins G (1993) Immunohistochemical study of intimal microvessels in coronary atherosclerosis. Am J Pathol 143:164–172
9. Capron L (1996) Évolution des théories sur l'athérosclérose. Rev Prat (Paris) 46:533–537
10. Huchard H (1891) Les causes de l'artério-sclérose et des cardiopathies artérielles. Rev Gén Clin Thérap 5:637–639
11. Vallance P, Collier J, Bhagat K (1997) Infection, inflammation, and infarction: does acute endothelial dysfunction provide a link? Lancet 349:1391–1392
12. Wick G, Schett G, Amberger A, Kleindienst R, Xu QB (1995) Is atherosclerosis an immunologically mediated disease? Immunol Today 16:27–33
13. Capron L (1996) Chlamydia in coronary plaques – Hidden culprit or harmless hobo? Nature Med 2:856–857
14. Danesh J, Collins R, Peto R (1997) Chronic infections and coronary heart disease: is there a link? Lancet 350:430–436
15. Fabricant CG, Fabricant J, Litrenta MM, Minick CR (1978) Virus-induced atherosclerosis. J Exp Med 148:335–340
16. Nicholson AC, Hajjar DP (1998) Herpesviruses in atherosclerosis and thrombosis: Etiologic agents or ubiquitous bystanders? Arterioscler Thromb Vasc Biol 18:339–348
17. Hendrix MGR, Salimans MMM, Vanboven CPA, Bruggeman CA (1990) High prevalence of latently present cytomegalovirus in arterial walls of patients suffering from grade-III atherosclerosis. Am J Pathol 136:23–28
18. Gag SZ, Hunt SA, Schroeder JS, Alderman EL, Hill IR, Stinson EB (1996) Early development of accelerated graft coronary artery disease: Risk factors and course. J Am Coll Cardiol 28:673–679
19. Wu TC, Hruban RH, Ambinder RF, et al. (1992) Demonstration of cytomegalovirus nucleic acids in the coronary arteries of transplanted hearts. Am J Pathol 140:739–747
20. Gulizia JM, Kandolf R, Kendall TJ, et al. (1995) Infrequency of cytomegalovirus genome in coronary arteriopathy of human heart allografts. Am J Pathol 147:461–475
21. Zhou YF, Leon MB, Waclawiw MA, et al. (1996) Association between prior cytomegalovirus infection and the risk of restenosis after coronary atherectomy. N Engl J Med 335:624–630
22. Speir E, Modali R, Huang ES, et al. (1994) Potential role of human cytomegalovirus and p53 interaction in coronary restenosis. Science 265:391–394
23. Blum A, Giladi M, Weinberg M, et al. (1998) High anti-cytomegalovirus (CMV) IgG antibody titer is associated with coronary artery disease and may predict post-coronary balloon angioplasty restenosis. Am J Cardiol 81:866–868
24. Carlsson J, Miketic S, Mueller KH, et al. (1997 & 1998) Previous cytomegalovirus or Chlamydia pneumoniae infection and risk of restenosis after percutaneous transluminal coronary angioplasty. Lancet 350:1225 & 351:143 [letters].
25. Legrand A, Mayer EP, Dalvi SS, Nachtigal M (1997) Transformation of rabbit vascular smooth muscle cells by human cytomegalovirus morphological transforming region 1. Am J Pathol 151:1387–1395
26. Grayston JT, Kuo CC, Wang SP, Altman J (1986) A new Chlamydia psittaci strain, TWAR, isolated in acute respiratory track infections. N Engl J Med 315:161–168
27. Kuo CC, Jackson LA, Campbell LA, Grayston JT (1995) Chlamydia pneumoniae (TWAR). Clin Microbiol Rev 8:451–461

28. Saikku P, Leinonen M, Mattila K, et al. (1988) Serological evidence of an association of a novel Chlamydia, TWAR, with chronic coronary heart disease and acute myocardial infarction. Lancet ii:983–985

29. Moazed TC, Kuo CC, Patton DL, Grayston JT, Campbell LA (1996) Experimental rabbit models of Chlamydia pneumoniae infection. Am J Pathol 148:667–676

30. Moazed TC, Kuo CC, Grayston JT, Campbell LA (1997) Murine models of Chlamydia pneumoniae infection and atherosclerosis. J Infect Dis 175:883–890

31. Gaydos CA, Summersgill JT, Sahney NN, Ramirez JA, Quinn TC (1996) Replication of Chlamydia pneumoniae in vitro in human macrophages, endothelial cells, and aortic artery smooth muscle cells. Infect Immun 64:1614–1620

32. Molestina RE, Dean D, Miller RD, Ramirez JA, Summersgill JT (1998) Characterization of a strain of Chlamydia pneumoniae isolated from a coronary atheroma by analysis of the omp1 gene and biological activity in human endothelial cells. Infect Immun 66:1370–1376

33. Yamashita K, Ouchi K, Shirai M, Gondo T, Nakazawa T, Ito H (1998) Distribution of Chlamydia pneumoniae infection in the atherosclerotic carotid artery. Stroke 29:773–778

34. Danesh J, Peto R (1998) Risk factors for coronary heart disease and infection with Helicobacter pylori: meta-analysis of 18 studies. BMJ 316:1130–1132

35. Gupta S, Leatham EW, Carrington D, Mendall MA, Kaski JC, Camm AJ (1997) Elevated Chlamydia pneumoniae antibodies, cardiovascular events, and azithromycin in male survivors of myocardial infarction. Circulation 96:404–407

36. Gurfinkel E, Bozovich G, Daroca A, Beck E, Mautner B, for the ROXIS Study Group (1997) Randomised trial of roxithromycin in non-Q wave coronary syndromes: ROXIS pilot study. Lancet 350:404–407

37. Zhou YF, Guetta E, Yu ZX, Finkel T, Epstein SE (1996) Human cytomegalovirus increases modified low density lipoprotein uptake and scavenger receptor mRNA expression in vascular smooth muscle cells. J Clin Invest 98:2129–2138

Section II:
Applied Physiology

Myocardial Ischemic Preconditioning

D.M. Van Winkle

Introduction

Protection of ischemic myocardium through transient antecedent sublethal ischemia (myocardial ischemic preconditioning, IP) is a well established laboratory phenomenon which has caught the attention and imagination of clinicians and researchers throughout the world. The magnitude of protection against ischemic injury conferred by IP is tremendous, far surpassing that offered by past pharmacological therapies. Indirect evidence suggests that IP occurs in human hearts as well. But whether IP is a naturally occurring phenomenon in humans, or is relevant to the practice of clinical medicine, remains unclear.

A Brief Overview of Myocardial Ischemic Preconditioning

Myocardial IP was first described in 1986 by Murry and colleagues, who found that canine myocardium subjected to repetitive coronary occlusion and reperfusion exhibited little necrosis, even though an equivalent duration of continuous coronary occlusion resulted in marked infarction [1]. Subsequent laboratory studies have demonstrated the presence of IP in every animal species tested [2–8].

The original description of IP was a limitation of myocardial infarct size following acute coronary occlusion and reperfusion [1]. However, subsequent laboratory studies have shown that IP may also decrease the incidence of ischemia-induced arrhythmias and improve post-ischemic cardiac function [9–12]. Not all studies of IP have demonstrated improved post-ischemic contractile function in preconditioned hearts as compared to non-preconditioned hearts [13, 14]. However, this apparent discrepancy is likely model dependent: experimental models utilizing a sustained second ischemic period may result in some infarction. In such a case it is difficult to ascertain whether contractile dysfunction is due to loss of viable cells or due to dysfunction of reversibly injured myocytes. Further, positive reports of improved post-ischemic contractile function in preconditioned hearts have come largely from experimental preparations employing rat or rabbit hearts, whereas those studies not finding preserved improved post-ischemic contractile function in preconditioned hearts are mostly from experimental preparations employing larger animals such as dogs or pigs.

It is also important to realize that the cellular mechanisms responsible for the infarct limiting effect of IP may be different from those mechanisms responsible for IP-induced improved post-ischemic contractile function or decreased incidence of malignant arrhythmias. For instance, whereas the infarct limiting effect is strongly associated with activation of sarcolemmal A_1 adenosine receptors, the anti-arrhythmic effect of preconditioning is not adenosine-dependent [15].

Cardioprotection following transient sublethal ischemia occurs in two distinct time windows: acutely (minutes to ~ 2 h after preconditioning ischemia, "classical preconditioning") [16] and remote from the preconditioning stimulus (24–48 h after preconditioning ischemia, "second window of protection," SWOP, or "late preconditioning") [17]. As with the different endpoints of IP, the mechanism(s) responsible for classical preconditioning may be different from the mechanism(s) responsible for late preconditioning. Unless specifically stated, the remainder of this review will concentrate on classical IP.

The Natural History of Ischemic Preconditioning

The amount of ischemia necessary to elicit preconditioning varies among experimental preparations and species, but uniformly is of a few minutes duration. Anesthetized open chest dogs and rabbits are near maximally protected with a single 5-minute period of preconditioning ischemia [16]. In contrast, swine require 1–2 cycles of 10 min ischemia to elicit preconditioning, [2, 18, 19] and rodents may require multiple preconditioning cycles [4, 8, 20]. The minimal amount of ischemia human myocardium must undergo to become maximally preconditioned is currently unknown. Percutaneous transluminal angioplasty studies utilizing 90 s balloon inflations and showing presumptive IP suggest that the duration of ischemia required in humans may be quite short [21, 22]. However, a short duration of ischemia may cause sub-maximal expression of IP. Thus the duration of ischemia required for *optimal* preconditioning of human hearts is still unknown.

The window of time during which classical preconditioning limits infarct size dissipates gradually beginning at approximately 60 min after the preconditioning stimulus, and is virtually absent 120 min after the preconditioning stimulus [16, 23]. Preconditioning can be reinstituted after this protective window has elapsed by application of another cycle of preconditioning ischemia; however, chronically repetitive transient ischemic episodes (≥4 in the rabbit) do not protect and suggest a tachyphylaxis-like process [24–26]

Cellular Mechanisms of Ischemic Preconditioning

The mechanisms responsible for the protective effects IP are not fully understood. The initial step in triggering IP is the occupation and activation of certain sarcolemmal receptors by their endogeous ligands. Most notable among these are adenosine A_1 receptors, whose activation appears to be necessary during both the preconditioning ischemia and the subsequent longer ischemic episode [3, 27].

Other receptors that may participate in IP include α-adrenergic receptors, bradykinin B_2 receptors, and opioid receptors [28–31]. Additionally, oxygen free radicals generated during preconditioning ischemia/reperfusion participate in the initiation of IP [32]. All of the above are thought to elicit a kinase cascade, in which activated protein kinase C causes activation of a tyrosine kinase. The ultimate target of this kinase cascade is not known but likely involves the ATP-sensitive potassium channel (K_{ATP}), since blockade of this channel abolishes preconditioning [33–35]. Other possible targets include cytoskeletal structural proteins. Figure 1 presents a schematic overview of cellular mechanisms in IP. Signal transduction pathways in IP have been recently reviewed by Downey and Cohen [36].

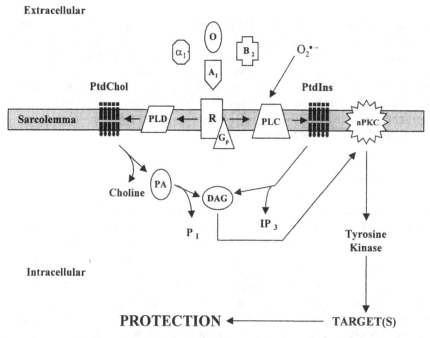

Fig. 1. Schematic diagram showing postulated cellular mechanisms responsible for the infarct-limiting effect of ischemic preconditioning. Shown is the cardiomyocyte sarcolemma and signalling pathways. Substances which are thought to elicit preconditioning (α_1 α_1-adrenergic agonists; A_1 adenosine A_1 agonists; B_2 bradykinin B_2 agonists; O opioid agonists) interact with their specific sarcolemmal receptor. These receptors, via a pertussis toxin sensitive G protein (G_p), activate either phospholipase C (*PLC*) or phospholipase D (*PLD*) to generate diacylglycerol (*DAG*), which in turn activates protein kinase C (*PKC*). Activated PKC is thought to then activate a tyrosine kinase, which phosphorylates an unknown target, resutling in protection. Oxygen radicals ($O_2\cdot^-$) produced upon reperfusion from preconditioning ischemia are also thought to initiate this protective kinase cascade. The end effector of preconditioning is not known, but may be the ATP-sensitive potassium channel, or a cardiomyocyte structural protein. *IP₃* Inositol triphosphate; *PA* phosphatidic acid; P_i inorganic phosphate; *PtdChol* phosphotidylcholine; *PtdIns* phosphotidylinositol; *R* receptor

Ischemic Preconditioning in Humans

Ischemic preconditioning has been shown to exist in all animal species examined (dogs, pigs, rats, rabbits, mice, ferrets, marmots) [2–8]. Definitive evidence that IP occurs in humans is difficult to obtain, given methodologic constraints associated with human research and the fact that the "gold-standard" for identifying classical preconditioning is a reduction of myocardial infarct size. There are several conditions in which human preconditioning has been presumptively demonstrated: "warm-up" angina, prodromal angina, percutaneous transluminal angioplasty (PTCA), cardiopulmonary bypass (CPB), and in vitro human tissue preparations.

"Warm-Up" Angina

"Warm-up" angina and "walk-through" angina refer to the phenomena wherein an individual experiences angina upon initial exertion but the angina disappears after cessation and resumption of exercise or during continued exercise [37]. Although these phenomena has been well known for several decades, its mechanism has remained elusive. One possible explanation is that ischemia associated with the initial episode of angina preconditions the myocardium against further or continued ischemia. The "warm-up" phenomenon and its potential relationship to IP has been recently reviewed [38].

Prodromal Angina

Prodromal, or preinfarction, angina has also been suggested to be a clinical manifestation of IP in humans. In two retrospective studies, angina preceding infarction was associated with preserved regional contractile function and decreased infarct size (assessed by CK MB release); because there was no evidence of collateral vessels this was interpreted as evidence of preconditioning [39, 40]. Earlier studies have also demonstrated improved post-infarction left ventricular function in patients who experienced preinfarction angina [41, 42].

However, some studies have shown that preinfarction angina adversely affects short-term hospital outcome [43, 44] or long-term outcome [45, 46]. In these studies either thrombolytic therapy was not administered and/or the incidence of baseline cardiac risk factors was higher in patients with preinfarction angina than those without. Thus a lack of a beneficial effect would be expected in non-reperfused infarcts even if preinfarction angina did precondition the myocardium, since IP can delay but not prevent necrosis. Additionally, prodromal angina is often associated with multivessel coronary artery disease; this, in concert with poorer baseline characteristics than patients without preinfarction angina, may contribute to poor long-term outcome.

Overall, the evidence suggests that prodromal angina may indeed precondition human myocardium, but that this beneficial effect may be somewhat masked by poorer long term outcome secondary to multivessel and/or complicated disease.

Angioplasty

Deutsch et al. were the first investigators to report that the second of two 90 s balloon inflations was associated with less anginal intensity, less ST segment shift, and lower myocardial lactate production despite no increase in great cardiac vein flow [21]. Others have replicated this finding, using ST segment shifts, anginal intensity, and/or ventricular function as endpoints [22, 47]. In these studies there were no angiographically visible collateral vessels; however, other investigators reporting adaptation to ischemia during PTCA have demonstrated collateral recruitment with sequential balloon inflations ($\geq$ 120 s each) [48]. Thus, in some but not all patients, PTCA-induced adaptation to ischemia may be due to enhanced collateral flow to the ischemic tissue.

Not all studies have reported a beneficial effect of PTCA on subsequent balloon inflations. For example, Dupouy et al. reported that in patients without angiographic evidence of collateral vessels, repeated balloon inflations did not provide any protection against ischemia, as assessed by ST-segment shifts and septal wall thickening (M-mode echocardiography) [49]. However, Bolli and colleagues argue that in the Dupouy study ST segments were measured too early (ST segments were measured at 90 s of a 120 s balloon inflation), and assert that "evidence of preconditioning has been found consistently in those studies that have recorded the ECG for 120 s... but inconsistently in those studies that have recorded the ECG for <120 s" [50].

Overall, evidence from PTCA studies suggests that the beneficial effects resulting from the initial balloon inflation are due to collateral recruitment in some patients, and a preconditioning-like adaptation in others.

Cardiac Surgery

The most obvious clinical arena where preconditioning might be utilized is cardiac surgery. There have been few clinical studies examining the potential for IP during cardiac surgery, and these have yielded differing results [51–56]. Perrault et al. failed to demonstrate enhanced protection by IP during cardiopulmonary bypass as opposed to retrograde cardioplegia alone [53]. However, it is not clear that in this setting the single 3 min period of aortic cross-clamping was sufficient to elicit the preconditioning phenomenon. We and others have shown that hypothermia during preconditioning ischemia increases the threshold for the amount of ischemia necessary to elicit cardiac protection [57, 58]. Since temperature in the Perrault et al. study was 31–32°C, an adequate ischemic stimulus to induce IP may not have been present. Additionally, assessment of protection was not performed after the termination of bypass. Kaukoranta et al. also failed to find augmented protection in hearts rendered ischemic for 5 min before arrest and normothermic retrograde cardioplegia [56]. Again, indices of protection were not measured after termination of bypass.

In contrast, the initial study examining IP in humans undergoing cardiopulmonary bypass showed that myocardium preconditioned with two 3-minute periods of aortic cross-clamping exhibited preserved ATP levels following 10 min of normothermic cross-clamping with electrical ventricular fibrillation, as compared to non-preconditioned hearts [51]. Using the same paradigm, Jenkins et al. demonstrated that serum troponin T levels were nearly 4-fold lower at 72 h postoperatively in preconditioned hearts as compared to non-preconditioned hearts [52]. Other studies, in which post-ischemic cardiac function was used to assess preconditioning, have found that IP protects human myocardium [54, 55]. Additionally, the need for inotropic support was greatly reduced in preconditioned patients [54].

Recently, the role of IP during minimally invasive coronary artery bypass surgery (MIDCAB) has begun to be evaluated. In a case presentation, it was reported that a MIDCAB performed with preconditioning provided a good outcome with good revascularization and no evidence of perioperative infarction [59]. However, this relevance of IP to the successful outcome in this case report is complicated by the use of esmolol. In contrast, protection was not found in hearts preconditioned with 5 min coronary artery occlusion, as assessed by transesophageal echocardiography during the subsequent grafting coronary artery occlusion [60]. However, a non-preconditioned control group was not included in the experimental design of this study, nor was function assessed following revascularization. In summary, based upon current data it is unclear whether IP can substantially improve outcome following MIDCAB, and this topic merits future investigation. The potential role of IP in cardiac surgery has been previously reviewed [61–64].

In Vitro Studies

In cultured quiescent human ventricular cardiomyocytes, IP reduced lactate dehydrogenase release, reduced cellular injury as assessed by trypan blue uptake, and increased the number of surviving cells following simulated ischemia [65]. Using isolated superfused contracting human right atrial trabeculae, Walker et al. demonstrated that tissue preconditioned by 3 min ischemia displayed improved post-ischemic contractile function as compared to non-preconditioned trabeculae [66]. Because there are functional differences between atrial and ventricular tissue, these results must be extrapolated to ventricular tissue with caution. However, a subsequent report noted similar functional protection from IP in human ventricular trabeculae [67]. Overall, the observation that transient antecedent simulated ischemia is protective two different in vitro preparations suggests human myocardium can be preconditioned.

Mechanisms of IP in Humans

Not surprisingly, many of the mediators that participate in IP in non-human species also appear to participate in IP in humans. Adenosine receptors, α-adrenergic receptors, and bradykinin B_2 receptors have all been shown to mediate IP in human isolated superfused cardiac trabeculae [66, 68, 69]. Additionally, activation of K_{ATP} channels also appears to be a key event in human IP [70, 71].

Preconditioning in the Presence of Pathologic Conditions

Typically, studies of preconditioning involving laboratory animals are performed on a select group of like animals that do not exhibit ongoing pathology. However, disease affects many human patients with cardiovascular disease, and may alter their response to IP.

Hypertrophy

Cardiac hypertrophy is common in the patient population for whom IP is of particular importance. Speechly-Dick et al. demonstrated preserved IP-induced infarct limitation in hypertrophied myocardium from rats with mineralocorticoid-induced hypertension [72]. Subsequently, it was shown that IP can improve post-ischemic cardiac function in isolated hearts from spontaneously hypertensive rats [73]. Recently, it has been reported that isolated hearts from transgenic [mREN-2)27] hypertensive rats, perfused at constant flow to eliminate the impaired post-ischemic hyperemia associated with hypertrophied myocardium, exhibit *enhanced* preconditioning-induced recovery of function as compared to normotensive controls [74]. Together, these data strongly show that IP is preserved in hypertension-induced myocardial hypertrophy.

Diabetes

Recently, it was reported that diabetic patients without previous myocardial infarction have as high a risk of myocardial infarction as non-diabetic patients with previous myocardial infarction, [75] likely due to accelerated atherosclerosis. However, in experimentally induced regional myocardial ischemia and reperfusion, hearts from rats with streptozotocin-induced non-insulin-dependent diabetes (NIDD) display smaller infarcts than hearts from healthy controls, suggesting that NIDD protects the heart from infarction once coronary flow is impeded [76].

Recently, it has been suggested that patients taking oral hypoglycemic agents of the sulfonylurea class may actually be at risk for exacerbated myocardial damage during ischemic events [77]. The primary anti-diabetic action of sulfonylureas is stimulation of insulin release by blockade of pancreatic β-cell K_{ATP} channels. Sulfonylureas also cause the release of certain membrane anchored proteins such as ecto-5'-nucleotidase. However, blockade of K_{ATP} channels in myocardium is associated with abolition of IP, and loss of ecto-5'-nucleotidase could potentially reduce adenosine concentration near the sarcolemmal adenosine receptor. These effects could worsen the impact of acute myocardial ischemia.

Cleveland et al. examined this question using isolated superfused atrial trabeculae [78]. They found that preconditioned trabeculae from diabetics taking oral sulfonylureas had a significantly lower post-ischemic recovery of developed force than preconditioned trabeculae from diabetics taking insulin or non-diabetic individuals. Additionally, recovery of developed force in preconditioned trabeculae from diabetics taking oral sulfonylureas was not different from non-preconditioned trabeculae from non-diabetics. Although it is premature to alter clinical practice based upon this one study, clearly these data suggest that diabetic therapy may have an important influence on recovery from myocardial ischemia.

Other Clinically Used Agents and Preconditioning

We noted that there was a marked variation in the reported magnitude of preconditioning protection in laboratory animal studies, and that these studies used a variety of anesthetic agents. We examined whether anesthetic choice alters preconditioning and found that among the commonly used veterinary anesthetics pentobarbital, ketamine/xylazine cocktail, and isoflurane, protection from IP varied widely [79]. isoflurane Additionally, there was a (non-significant) trend for isoflurane-anesthetized animals to display smaller infarcts than those anesthetized with ketamine/xylazine or pentobarbital. Subsequently, Cope et al. reported a significant decrease in infarct size with isoflurane anesthetized rabbits as compared to pentobarbital, ketamine/xylazine, or propofol [80].

Volatile anesthetics have also been examined in preconditioning paradigms. In isolated rat hearts, both isoflurane and halothane increased post-ischemic recovery of left ventricular developed pressure in a manner that was equipotent with IP [81]. Administration of these volatile agents in addition to IP did not elicit any further protection. However, it is possible that the IP stimulus given provided maximal protection; whether protection from a sub-maximal IP stimulus can be augmented by volatile anesthetics was not addressed in this study. These results were confirmed and extended to include enflurane by Cope et al. who showed a decrease in infarct size by all three agents in isolated rabbit hearts, equipotent with IP [80]. Halothane-induced infarct limitation was abolished by adenosine receptor blockade and protein kinase C blockade, both of which appear to participate in signal transduction in IP.

Similarly, in barbiturate anesthetized dogs, 1 MAC isoflurane limited infarct size in a manner equipotent with IP. However, these investigators found that the combination of IP and isoflurane provided even further reductions of infarct size. Additionally, it was found that the sulfonylurea glibenclamide abolished isoflurane-induced protection; thus it was concluded that, like IP, isoflurane-induced protection involves K_{ATP} channels [82]. In propofol anesthetized rabbits, ~0.5 MAC isoflurane decreased infarct size, but the protective effect of isoflurane was much smaller than that seen with IP [83]. Whether this difference was due to the amount of isoflurane used (0.5 MAC vs 1 MAC in the Kersten et al. study) or the amount of protection provided by IP (74% decrease in infarct size vs 62% in the Kersten et al. study) cannot be ascertained from these studies.

Gross and co-workers examined the effect of narcotic antagonists and agonists on IP and ischemic damage. They found that in pentobarbital anesthetized rats 3 mg/kg iv naloxone completely abolished the infarct limiting effect of IP, [29] and that 300 µg/kg iv morphine limited infarct size equipotent with IP [84]. Morphine-induced protection was blocked by the sulfonylurea glyburide, which also abolishes IP. Subsequently, we confirmed Gross' findings and extended them by finding that naloxone blockade of IP (a) occurs in rabbits as well as rats, and (b) is stereoselective [85].

The opioid receptor subtype(s) and opioid peptide(s) involved in IP are not yet fully described. However, pharmacologic evidence suggests that the δ opioid receptor is a likely candidate [86, 87]. Transgenic mice deficient in endogenous β-endorphin exhibit IP, suggesting that this opioid peptide is not the sole endogenous opioid which participates in IP [88].

Together, all these studies show that the choice of anesthetic/analgesic can exert a profound effect on myocardial damage during acute myocardial ischemia and reperfusion, both in the absence and presence of IP.

Summary and Conclusions

The magnitude of protection that IP confers against experimentally induced myocardial ischemia-reperfusion is substantial. Whether this endogenous protective phenomenon operates naturally in humans is not yet clear, although there is considerable indirect clinical evidence indicating that preconditioning does occur naturally in humans. There is now ample laboratory evidence demonstrating that excised samples of human myocardium can be experimentally preconditioned. The impact of IP in the clinical and surgical arenas is only now beginning to be felt, and much work remains to be done to optimally implement our knowledge of preconditioning and preconditioning-mimetic agents into the clinical setting.

References

1. Murry CE, Jennings RB, and Reimer KA (1986) Preconditioning with ischemia: a delay of lethal cell injury in ischemic myocardium. Circulation, 74:1124–1136
2. Schott RJ, Rohmann S, Braun ER, and Schaper W (1990) Ischemic preconditioning reduces infarct size in swine myocardium. Circ Res, 66:1133–1142
3. Liu GS, Thornton J, Van Winkle DM, Stanley AWH, Olsson RA, and Downey JM (1991) Protection against infarction afforded by preconditioning is mediated by A1 adenosine receptors in rabbit heart. Circulation, 84:350–356
4. Liu Y and Downey JM (1992) Ischemic preconditioning protects against infarction in rat heart. Am J Physiol, 263:H1107-H1112
5. Li GC, Vasquez JA, Gallagher KP, and Lucchesi BR (1989) Ischemic preconditioning requires only one, five minute coronary artery occlusion. Circulation, 80:II-240 (Abstract)
6. Gomoll AW (1996) Cardioprotection associated with preconditioning in the anesthetized ferret. Basic Res Cardiol, 91:433–443
7. McKean T and Mendenhall W (1996) Comparison of the responses to hypoxia, ischaemia and ischaemic preconditioning in wild marmot and laboratory rabbit hearts. J Exp Biol, 199:693–697
8. Miller DL, Wolff RA, and Van Winkle DM (1998) Ischemic preconditioning in murine myocardium. FASEB J, 12:A75 (Abstract)
9. Shiki K and Hearse DJ (1987) Preconditioning of ischemic myocardium: reperfusion-induced arrhythmias. Am J Physiol, 253:H1470-H1476

10. Vegh A, Komori S, Szekeres L, and Parratt JR (1992) Antiarrhythmic effects of preconditioning in anesthetized dogs and rats. Cardiovasc Res, 26:487–495

11. Cave AC (1995) Preconditioning induced protection against post-ischaemic contractile dysfunction: characteristics and mechanisms. J Mol Cell Cardiol, 27:969–979

12. Cohen MV, Liu GS, and Downey JM (1991) Preconditioning causes improved wall motion as well as smaller infarcts after transient coronary occlusion in rabbits. Circulation, 84:341–349.

13. Ovize M, Przyklenk K, Hale SL, and Kloner RA (1992) Preconditioning does not attenuate myocardial stunning. Circulation, 85:2247–2254

14. Miyamae M, Fujiwara H, Kida M, et al. (1993) Preconditioning improves energy metabolism during reperfusion but does not attenuate myocardial stunning in porcine hearts. Circulation, 88:223–234

15. Vegh A, Papp JG, and Parratt JR (1995) Pronounced antiarrhythmic effects of preconditioning in anaesthetized dogs: is adenosine involved? J Mol Cell Cardiol, 27:349–356

16. Van Winkle DM, Thornton J, Downey DM, and Downey JM (1991) The natural history of preconditioning. Cardioprotection depends on duration of transient ischemia and time to subsequent ischemia. Cor Art Dis, 2:613–619

17. Baxter GF, Marber MS, Patel VC, and Yellon DM (1994) Adenosine receptor involvement in a delayed phase of myocardial protection 24 h after ischemic preconditioning. Circulation, 90:2993–3000

18. Schulz R, Rose J, Post H, and Heusch G (1995) Involvement of endogenous adenosine in ischaemic preconditioning in swine. Pflügers Arch, 430:273–282

19. Van Winkle DM, Chien GL, Wolff RA, and Davis RD (1992) Intracoronary infusion of R-phenylisopropyl adenosine prior to ischemia/reperfusion reduces myocardial infarct size in swine. Circulation, 86 (4):I-213 (Abstract)

20. Yellon DM, Alkhulaifi AM, Browne EE, and Pugsley WB (1992) Ischaemic preconditioning limits infarct size in the rat heart. Cardiovasc Res, 26:983–987

21. Deutsch E, Berger M, Kussmaul WG, Hirshfeld JW, Jr., Herrmann H, and Laskey WK (1991) Adaptation to ischemia during percutaneous transluminal coronary angioplasty. Clinical, hemodynamic, and metabolic features. Circulation, 82:2044–2051

22. Inoue T, Fujito T, Hoshi K, et al. (1996) A mechanism of ischemic preconditioning during percutaneous transluminal coronary angioplasty. Cardiol, 87:216–223

23. Miura T and Iimura O (1993) Infarct size limitation by preconditioning: its phenomenological features and the key role of adenosine. Cardiovasc Res, 27:36–42

24. Cohen MV, Yang X-M, and Downey JM (1994) Conscious rabbits become tolerant to multiple episodes of ischemic preconditioning. Circ Res, 74:998–1004

25. Yang X-M, Arnoult S, Tsuchida A, et al. (1993) The protection of ischemic preconditioning can be reinstated in the rabbit heart after the initial protection has waned. Cardiovasc Res, 27:556–558

26. Iliodromitis EK, Kremastinos DTh, Katritsis DG, Papadopoulos CC, and Hearse DJ (1997) Multiple cycles of preconditioning cause loss of protection in open-chest rabbits. J Mol Cell Cardiol, 29:915–920

27. Thornton JD, Thornton CS, and Downey JM (1993) Effect of adenosine receptor blockade: preventing protective preconditioning depends on time of initiation. Am J Physiol, 265:H504-H508

28. Wall TM, Sheehy R, and Hartman JC (1994) Role of bradykinin in myocardial preconditioning. J Pharmacol Exp Ther, 270:681–688

29. Schultz JEJ, Rose E, Yao Z, and Gross GJ (1995) Evidence for involvement of opioid receptors in ischemic preconditioning in rat hearts. Am J Physiol, 268:H2157-H2161

30. Banerjee A, Locke-Winter C, Rogers KB, et al. (1993) Preconditioning against myocardial dysfunction after ischemia and reperfusion by an α1-adrenergic mechanism. Circ Res, 73:656–670

31. Kitakaze M, Hori M, Morioka T, et al. (1994) α1-Adrenoceptor activation mediates the infarct size-limiting effect of ischemic preconditioning through augmentation of 5'-nucleotidase activity. J Clin Invest, 95:2197–2205

32. Ambrosio G, Tritto I, and Chiariello M (1995) The role of oxygen free radicals in preconditioning. J Mol Cell Cardiol, 27:1035–1039
33. Gross GJ and Auchampach JA (1992) Blockade of ATP-sensitive potassium channels prevents myocardial preconditioning in dogs. Circ Res, 70:223–233
34. Schulz R, Rose J, and Heusch G (1994) Involvement of activation of ATP-dependent potassium channels in ischemic preconditioning in swine. Am J Physiol, 267:H1341–H1352
35. Miura T, Goto M, Miki T, Sakamoto J, Shimamoto K, and Iimura O (1995) Glibenclamide, a blocker of ATP-sensitive potassium channels, abolishes infarct size limitation by preconditioning in rabbits anesthetized with xylazine/pentobarbital but not with pentobarbital alone. J Cardiovasc Pharmacol, 25:531–538
36. Downey JM and Cohen MV (1997) Signal transduction in ischemic preconditioning. Adv Exp Med Biol, 430:39–55
37. Kloner RA and Yellon DM (1994) Does ischemic preconditioning occur in patients? J Am Coll Cardiol, 24:1133–1142
38. Marber MS, Joy MD, and Yellon DM (1994) Is warm-up angina ischaemic preconditioning? Br Heart J, 72:213–214
39. Ottani F, Galvani M, Ferrini D, et al. (1995) Prodromal angina limits infarct size: A role for ischemic preconditioning. Circulation, 91:291–297
40. Nakagawa Y, Ito H, Kitakaze M, et al. (1995) Effect of angina pectoris on myocardial protection in patients with reperfused anterior wall myocardial infarction: retrospective clinical evidence of "preconditioning". J Am Coll Cardiol, 25:1076–1083
41. Cortina A, Ambrose JA, Prieto-Granada J, and et al. (1985) Left ventricular function after myocardial infarction: clinical and angiographic correlates. J Am Coll Cardiol, 5:619–624
42. Matsuda Y, Ogawa H, Moritani K, and et al. (1984) Effects of the presence or absence of preceding angina pectoris on left ventricular function after acute myocardial infarction. Am Heart J, 108:955–958
43. Barbash GI, White HD, Modan M, Van de Werf F, and et al. (1992) Antecedent angina pectoris predicts worse outcome after myocardial infarction in patients receiving thrombolytic therapy: experience gleaned from the International Tissue Plasminogen Activator/Streptokinase Mortality Trial. J Am Coll Cardiol, 20:36–41
44. Behar S, Reicher RH, Abinader E, and et al. (1992) The prognostic significance of angina pectoris preceding the occurrence of a first acute myocardial infarction in 4166 consecutive hospitalized patients. Am Heart J, 123:1481–1486
45. Harper RW, Kennedy G, DeSanctis RW, and Hutter AM, Jr. (1979) The incidence and pattern of angina prior to acute myocardial infarction: a study of 577 cases. Am Heart J, 79:178–183
46. Cupples IA, Gagnon DR, Wong ND, Ostfeld AM, and Kannel WB (1993) Pre-existing cardiovascular conditions and long-term prognosis after initial myocardial infarction: the Framingham study. Am Heart J, 125:863–872
47. Leesar MA, Stoddard M, Ahmed M, Broadbent J, and Bolli R (1997) Preconditioning of human myocardium with adenosine during coronary angioplasty. Circulation, 95:2500–2507
48. Cribier A, Korsatz L, Koning R, et al. (1992) Improved myocardial ischemic response and enhanced collateral circulation with long repetitive coronary occlusion during angioplasty: a prospective study. J Am Coll Cardiol, 20:578–586
49. Dupouy P, Geschwind H, Pelle G, et al. (1996) Repeated coronary artery occlusions during routine balloon angioplasty do not induce myocardial preconditioning in humans. J Am Coll Cardiol, 27:1374–1380
50. Bolli R, Leesar MA, and Stoddard M (1997) Ischemic preconditioning during coronary angioplasty. J Am Coll Cardiol, 29:469–470
51. Yellon DM, Alkhulaifi AM, and Pugsley WB (1993) Preconditioning the human myocardium. Lancet, 342:276–277
52. Jenkins DP, Pugsley WB, Alkhulaifi AM, Kemp M, Hooper J, and Yellon DM (1997) Ischaemic preconditioning reduces troponin T release in patients undergoing coronary artery bypass surgery. Heart, 77:314–318

53. Perrault LP, Menashé P, Bel A, et al. (1996) Ischemic preconditioning in cardiac surgery: a word of caution. J Thorac Cardiovasc Surg, 112:1378–1386

54. Illes RW and Swoyer KD (1998) Prospective, randomized clinical study of ischemic preconditioning as an adjunct to intermittent cold blood cardioplegia. Ann Thorac Surg, 65:748–753

55. Lu E-X, Chen S-X, Yuan M-D, et al. (1997) Preconditioning improves myocardial preservation in patients undergoing open heart operations. Ann Thorac Surg, 64:1320–1324

56. Kaukoranta PK, Lepojärvi MPK, Ylitalo KV, Kiviluoma KT, and Peuhkurinen KJ (1997) Normothermic retrograde blood cardioplegia with or without preceding ischemic preconditioning. Ann Thorac Surg, 63:1268–1274

57. Dote K, Wolff RA, and Van Winkle DM (1998) Hypothermia increases the threshold for ischemic preconditioning. J Thorac Cardiovasc Surg, 116:319–326

58. Lu E-X, Ying G-L, and Guo X (1997) Hypothermia during preconditioned ischemia-reperfusion attenuates the myocardial protection of preconditioning. J Thorac Cardiovasc Surg, 114:514–516

59. Jacobsohn E, Young CJ, Aronson S, Ferdinand FD, and Albertucci M (1998) Case 4–1997. The role of ischemic preconditioning during minimally invasive coronary artery bypass surgery. J Cardiothorac Vasc Anesth, 11:787–792

60. Malkowski MJ, Kramer CM, Parvizi ST, et al. (1998) Transient ischemia does not limit subsequent ischemic regional dysfunction in humans: a transesophageal echocardiographic study during minimally invasive coronary artery bypass surgery. J Am Coll Cardiol, 31: 1035–1039

61. Lasley RD and Mentzer RM (1995) Preconditioning and its potential role in myocardial protection during cardiac surgery. J Card Surg, 10:349–353

62. Kloner RA, Przyklenk K, Shook T, et al. (1995) Clinical aspects of preconditioning and implications for the cardiac surgeon. J Card Surg, 10:369–375

63. Alkhulaifi AM, Jenkins DP, Pugsley WB, and Treasure T (1996) Ischaemic preconditioning and cardiac surgery. Eur J Cardiothorac Surg, 10:792–798

64. Perrault LP and Menasché P (1997) Role of preconditioning in cardiac surgery. Basic Res Cardiol, 92:54–56

65. Ikonomidis JS, Tumiati LC, Weisel RD, Mickle DAG, and Li R-K (1994) Preconditioning human ventricular cardiomyocytes with brief periods of simulated ischaemia. Cardiovasc Res, 28:1285–1291

66. Walker DM, Walker JM, Pugsley WB, Pattison CW, and Yellon DM (1995) Preconditioning in isolated superfused human muscle. J Mol Cell Cardiol, 27 (6):1349–1357

67. Cleveland JC, Jr., Wollmering MM, Meldrum DR, et al. (1996) Ischemic preconditioning in human and rat ventricle. Am J Physiol, 271:H1786–H1794

68. Cleveland JC, Jr., Meldrum DR, Rowland RT, et al. (1997) Ischemic preconditioning of human myocardium: protein kinase C mediates a permissive role for α_1-adrenoceptors. Am J Physiol, 273:H902–H908

69. Morris SD and Yellon DM (1997) Angiotensin-converting enzyme inhibitors potentiate preconditioning through bradykinin B_2 receptor activation in human heart. J Am Coll Cardiol, 29:1599–1606

70. Carr CS, Grover GJ, Pugsley WB, and Yellon DM (1997) Comparison of the protective effects of a highly selective ATP-sensitive potassium channel opener and ischemic preconditioning in isolated human atrial muscle. Cardiovasc Drugs Ther, 11:473–478

71. Speechly-Dick ME, Grover GJ, and Yellon DM (1995) Does ischemic preconditioning in the human involve protein kinase C and the ATP-dependent K+ channel? Studies of contractile function after simulated ischemia in an atrial in vitro model. Circ Res, 77:1030–1035

72. Speechly-Dick ME, Baxter GF, and Yellon DM (1994) Ischaemic preconditioning protects hypertrophied myocardium. Cardiovasc Res, 28:1025–1029

73. Boutros A and Wang J (1995) Ischemic preconditioning, adenosine and bethanechol protect spontaneously hypertensive isolated rat hearts. The Journal of Pharmacology and Experimental Therapeutics, 2758:1148–1156

74. Randall MD, Gardiner SM, and Bennett T (1997) Enhanced cardiac preconditioning in the isolated heart of the transgenic ((mREN-2)27) hypertensive rat. Cardiovasc Res, 33:400–409
75. Haffner SM, Lehto S, Rönnemaa T, Pyörälä K, and Laakso M (1998) Mortality from coronary heart disease in subjects with type 2 diabetes and in non-diabetic subjects with and without prior myocardial infarction. N Engl J Med, 339:229–234
76. Liu Y, Thornton JD, Cohen MV, Downey JM, and Schaffer SW (1993) Streptozotocin-induced non-insulin-dependent diabetes protects the heart from infarction. Circulation, 88:1273–1278
77. Engler RL and Yellon DM (1996) Sulfonylurea K_{ATP} blockade in type II diabetes and preconditioning in cardiovascular disease. Time for reconsideration. Circulation, 94:2297–2301
78. Cleveland JC, Jr., Meldrum DR, Cain BS, Banerjee A, and Harken AH (1997) Oral sulfonylurea hypoglycemic agents prevent ischemic preconditioning in human myocardium. Two paradoxes revisited. Circulation, 96:29–32
79. Haessler R, Kuzume K, Chien GL, Wolff RA, Davis RF, and Van Winkle DM (1994) Anaesthetics alter the magnitude of infarct limitation by ischaemic preconditioning. Cardiovasc Res, 28:1574–1580
80. Cope DK, Impastato WK, Cohen MV, and Downey JM (1997) Volatile anesthetics protect the ischemic rabbit myocardium from infarction. Anesthesiology, 86:699–709
81. Boutros A, Wang J, and Capuano C (1997) Isoflurane and halothane increase adenosine triphosphate preservation, but do not provide additive recovery of function after ischemia, in preconditioned rat hearts. Anesthesiology, 86:109–117
82. Kersten JR, Schmeling TJ, Pagel PS, Gross GJ, and Warltier DC (1997) Isoflurane mimics ischemic preconditioning via activation of K_{ATP} channels. Anesthesiology, 87:361–370
83. Cason BA, Gamperl AK, Slocum RE, and Hickey RF (1997) Anesthetic-induced preconditioning: prevoius administration of isoflurane decreases myocardial infarct size in rabbits. Anesthesiology, 87:1182–1190
84. Schultz JEJ, Hsu AK, and Gross GJ (1996) Morphine mimics the cardioprotective effect of ischemic preconditioning via a glibenclamide-sensitive mechanism in rat heart. Circ Res, 78:1100–1104
85. Chien GL and Van Winkle DM (1996) Naloxone blockade of myocardial ischaemic preconditioning is stereoselective. J Mol Cell Cardiol, 28:1895–1900
86. Schultz JEJ, Hsu AK, and Gross GJ (1998) Ischemic preconditioning in the intact rat heart is mediated by δ_1- but not μ- or κ-opioid receptors. Circulation, 97:1282–1289
87. Schultz JEJ, Hsu AK, Nagase H, and Gross GJ (1998) TAN-67, a δ_1-opioid receptor agonist, reduces infarct size via activation of $G_{i/o}$ proteins and K_{ATP} channels. Am J Physiol, 274: H909-H914
88. Van Winkle, D.M., Miller, D.L., and Low, M.J. (1998): β-endorphin knock-out mice exhibit myocardial ischemic preconditioning. Circulation, 98 (17):I-416 (Abstract)

Coronary Circulation in Sepsis

J.-F. Dhainaut, N. Marin and J.D. Chiche

Introduction

Septic shock is characterized by increased cardiac output and diminished systemic vascular resistance, associated with widespread alterations of the circulatory control of tissue oxygen delivery. Microcirculatory dysfunction, hyporesponsiveness of arterial vessels, and depressed myocardial function have been identified in this syndrome. Indeed, strong evidence has also accumulated for myocardial dysfunction early in septic shock, even in the presence of an elevated cardiac output. Numerous studies have investigated the myocardial function in septic shock, but few investigations have coupled it to changes in coronary circulation, and its was suggested that inadequate coronary blood flow could play a role in the precipitation of heart dysfunction.

The Coronary Vasculature

Coronary blood flow in normal basal conditions is 80 ml/min/100 g. To meet the variable needs of the active myocardium, it is capable of increasing flow five-fold. With a normal arterial oxygen content, myocardial oxygen delivery varies between 15 and 50 ml/min/100 g. Myocardial oxygen extraction is thus 65–75%, a near maximal value in basal conditions. To achieve this high extraction, the myocardium possesses a rich capillary network, three to four times denser that skeletal muscle.

Extravascular forces directly influence coronary artery resistances and account for 30–40% of total resistance. Indeed, direct transmission of intraventricular pressures, by diminishing transmural pressures of coronary vessels, render the subendocardial layers particularly vulnerable to decreased coronary perfusion pressures. In addition, systolic ventricular torsion also affects total coronary resistances, such that systolic flow within the myocardium is zero, if not negative. Because of increased cell shortening and greater wall stress in the subendocardium, MVO_2 is 20% higher than in the subepicardial layers, explaining why flow is 20% to 40% higher in these layers.

Regulation of Myocardial Oxygen Delivery

In the isolated heart, coronary flow remains constant over a wide range of perfusing pressures: between 65–130 mmHG. With increased MVO_2 or decreased arterial oxygen content, coronary flow is augmented with higher but narrower autoregulatory flow plateau reflecting some loss of flow reserve. At maximal coronary vasodilation, flow becomes a linear increasing function of perfusion pressure. In vivo, however, all variations of perfusing pressure necessarily reflect changes in the external work of the heart, hence MVO_2, so that autoregulation occurs in the setting of an integrated response. An acute increase of the arterial blood pressure leads to an increased oxygen demand with consequent vasodilation of the coronary vascular bed, while autoregulation will limit pressure-induced flow. Flow-dependent vasodilation has been linked to the release of nitric oxide.

The importance of humoral control mechanisms in the regulation of myocardial O_2 delivery (MDO_2) has been emphasized, particularly in the setting of an altered endothelium. Many humoral substances (catecholamines, angiotensin, vasopressin thromboxane, prostacyclin, serotonin, etc.) exert significant direct effects on coronary vascular resistance, but most are indirect through altered ventricular work, in turn modifying metabolic requirements of the heart. Metabolic control is probably the predominant regulatory mechanism. The high turnover of ATP and its relatively low reserve imply that coronary oxygen transport bc tightly linked to metabolic requirements, and the near maximal extraction equates this with parallel variations of coronary blood flow (CBF). There is a linear relationship between MVO_2 and CBF. All variations of perfusion pressures necessarily translate parallel changes in the heart's loading conditions: decreased diastolic pressure diminishes left ventricular work, hence MVO_2.

Under physiologic conditions, coronary blood flow in proportion to the myocardial oxygen demand and the rate of myocardial oxygen consumption are closely related to the work performed. The ration oxygen consumption/oxygen delivery (oxygen extraction) is already at near maximal levels in normal conditions. All variations of systemic oxygen delivery because of altered loading conditions will change myocardial oxygen consumption. Coronary flow reserve, in the absence of stenotic lesions, enables the heart to face a wide range of systemic oxygen transport, as well as to meet myocardial oxygen demand. When compensatory mechanisms have been exhausted, the heart finds itself in critical conditions, for a 10–20% reduction of myocardial oxygen delivery by anemia, hypoxemia or reduced coronary blood flow suffices to induce myocardial dysfunction.

Human Septic Shock Studies

It was important to determine whether myocardial dysfunction in sepsis was due to an unrecognized hypoxia, especially in view of the altered oxygen extraction found present in peripheral organs and the elevated myocardial oxygen demand.

To test this hypothesis, Cunnion et al. (1986) compared coronary sinus blood flow in seven septic patients with subjects with normal coronary arteries at rest and during pacing. No significant differences were noted in coronary flow at heart rates below 100 beats/min. At heart rates above 100 beats/min, septic patients had higher coronary sinus blood flow than paced normal subjects. All patients had net myocardial lactate extraction. No correlation was observed in four patients with myocardial depression, coronary flow, and the net myocardial lactate extraction.

Conversely, Dhainaut et al. (1987) studied and compared 40 patients in septic shock with 13 control patients. The global hemodynamic pattern of the septic patients was characterized by a low stroke volume despite an elevated cardiac output. Coronary sinus blood flow was again higher in septic patients than in the control group due to marked coronary vasodilation (Fig. 1), while MVO_2, myocardial work loads and myocardial efficiency were not significantly different in the control and septic patients. Under physiologic conditions, coronary blood flow changes in proportion to the myocardial oxygen demand and the rate of myocardial oxygen consumption are closely related to the work performed. In this clinical study, coronary blood flow was higher in septic patients than in controls at any given workload, suggesting an unexplained marked coronary vasodilation. This apparently inappropriate high coronary blood flow in the septic patients may be due to several reasons. an inappropriate release of putative vasodilator substance (nitric oxide: NO) that would possibly result in a loss of auto-regulation, and a number of serum substances with the capacity to induce myocardial depression recently described in patients with sepsis might cause inappropriately high coro-

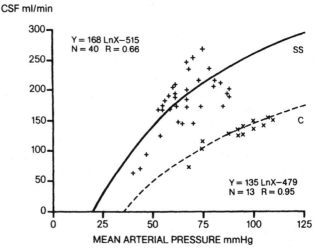

Fig. 1. Pressure-flow relationship in the patients with septic shock (*SS*) and the control group (*C*). Note that the pressure-flow relationship is curvilinear and the best fits a logarithmic equation. In patients with septic shock, the pressure-flow relationship is steeper and the zero-flow pressure intercept is lower than in control patients. *CSF* Coronary sinus blood flow. (From Dhainaut et al. 1987)

nary blood flow. An alteration in myocardial substrate extraction consisted of a depressed free fatty acids uptake and an increase uptake of lactate may also play a role (Fig. 2).

Only six of 40 septic patients with particularly low cardiac output and coronary perfusion pressure developed a myocardial ischemia (myocardial lactate production). The other 34 septic patients had a markedly high lactate extraction. However, lactate is a poor predictor of myocardial ischemia and it was therefore interesting to examine other biochemical markers of ischemia. Lowering of intracellular oxydoreduction potential leads to: decreased fatty acid catabolism secondary to accumulation of NADH, increased anaerobic glycosis, and increased rate of transamination reactions (quantitatively the most important being that of pyruvate by glutamate to yield α keto-glutarate and alanine). All six lactate producers also presented other biochemical signs of transition to an anaerobic metabolism, decreased free fatty acid consumption, increased consumption of glucose, and increased alanine production in association with a decreased MVO_2 (Table 1). Reestablishing coronary perfusion pressure with vasoactive agents led to increased CBF, and lactate was once again consumed by the myocardium.

Effects of Inotropic Support

In this study 10 patients had low cardiac index (<3.0 l/min/m²), and the administration of the combination of dobutamine and dopamine produced an increase in blood pressure, cardiac output, coronary sinus blood flow, MVO_2, and myocardial lactate uptake (Fig. 3). Thus, despite high levels of inotropic drugs, myocardial hypoxemia vanishes, because the increase in myocardial oxygen supply is higher than the increase in myocardial oxygen demand.

Six other patients had high cardiac index and low mean arterial pressure (<60 mmHG), dopamine infusion was followed by an increase in arterial pres-

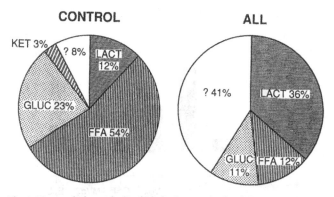

Fig. 2. Myocardial metabolic shift during septic shock. In comparison, patients with septic shock consume preferentially lactates, independently of their arterial concentrations. A substantial fraction of the energy source is unaccounted, suggesting consumption of endogenous energy supplies. *Lact* Lactate; *FFA* fatty free acids; *Gluc* glucose; *Ket* ketone bodies. (From Dhainaut et al. 1987)

Table 1. Myocardial metabolism was studied in 13 control patients undergoing cardiac catheterization for valvular heart disease and 40 patients with septic shock (*MAP*, mean arterial pressure, *CI* cardiac index, *MVO₂* myocardial oxygen consumption, *MextO₂* myocardial oxygen extraction, *CSF* coronary sinus flow, *Lact Cons* myocardial lactate consumption, *Ala Cons* myocardial alanine consumption, *Glut Cons* myocardial glutamate consumption, *Glu Cons* myocardial glucose consumption, *FFA Cons* myocardial free fatty acid consumption)

	Control (n=13)	Group 1 (n=34)	Group 2 (n=6)	Treatment (dopamine, dobutamine)
MAP (mmHG)	92±13	68±11[b]	50±8[d]	64±10[f]
CI (l/min/m²)	3.75±0.70	5.26±1.1	2.23±0.39[d]	4.35±0.41[f]
MVO₂ (ml/min)	15.5±1.6	16.7±3.8	8.9±4.0[d]	12.5±6.1[e]
MextO₂ (%)	67±7	50±5[b]	53±5	48±10
CBF (ml/min)	130±21	200±29[b]	109±37[d]	165±42[f]
Lact Cons (μmol/min)	20.3±6.5	73.6±47.3[b]	−17.3±12.7[d]	26.7±10.9[f]
Ala Cons (μmol/min)	−1.08±0.89	-2.0±2.2	−4.2±1.3[c]	−3.4±1.36
Glut Cons (μmol/min)	1.46±1.09	0.5±0.8[a]	1.1±0.4	0.5±1.9
Glu Cons (μmol/min)	20±6	9±6	14±5	–
FFA Cons (μmol/min)	12±3	3.0±5.9[b]	1.3±1.2	1.8±1.6

[a]$P<0.05$ between control and group 1, [b]$P<0.01$ between control and group 1, [c]$P<0.05$ between group 1 and group 2, [d]$P<0.01$ between group 1 and group 2, [e]$P<0.05$ between group 2 and group 2 after treatment with dopamine and dobutamine, [f]$P<0.01$ between group 2 and group 2 after treatment.

The unique myocardial metabolic profile has been previously reported. Biochemical signs of ischemia include myocardial lactate production, enhanced alanine production, increased glutamate extraction, and increased glucose consumption. A subgroup of six patients with low MAP, low CBF, and cardiac output were lactate producers. These six patients also demonstrated, while not always significant, other biochemical signs of ischemia.

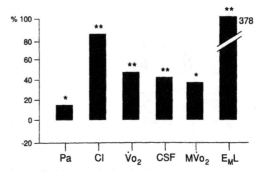

Fig. 3. Effects of the combination of dopamine and dobutamine in ten patients with low cardiac output induced by septic shock. *AP* Mean arterial pressure; *CI* cardiac index; *VO₂* systemic oxygen consumption; *CSF* coronary sinus blood flow; *MVO₂* myocardial oxygen consumption; *LU* myocardial lactate uptake. (From Schremmer and Dhainaut 1990)

sure, coronary sinus flow, MVO$_2$, and myocardial lactate uptake (Fig. 3). The other hemodynamic and metabolic parameters did not change. None of the six patients presented metabolic signs of myocardial hypoxemia before or after dopamine infusion. The beneficial effect of hemodynamic support is less obvious in these 6 patients than that obtained in the 10 patients with both low cardiac output and arterial pressure.

Finally, human septic shock is characterized by a marked coronary vasodilation (probably related to NO production), and apparently adequate MVO$_2$ associated with profound changes in myocardial substrates extraction. However, the precise relationship between coronary circulation and cardiac function remains to be clarified.

Recent Insights from Animal Models of Sepsis

Decreased Coronary Vascular Reserve

To test the hypothesis that metabolic regulation of myocardial oxygen delivery is significantly disturbed in hyperdynamic sepsis, Bloos et al. (1996) studied the response of coronary circulation and myocardial metabolism to hypoxia in sheep. They measured and compared myocardial blood flow and oxygen extraction in a cecal ligation and perforation group and control group during hypoxia, which both augmented heart work and depressed connective oxygen transport. The metabolic coupling between oxygen delivery and oxygen demand in the myocardium was demonstrated in this model. However, the extend to which septic coronary circulation was able to adjust to changes in the myocardial oxygen availability was depressed. A limited ability to increase both coronary blood flow and oxygen extraction may explain why the septic myocardium reached a point where its oxygen uptake was not sustainable at an earlier time that was evident in control sheep. Sepsis infringes on the coronary circulatory reserve available to match increases in myocardial oxygen needs with rapid and parallel increases in oxygen availability.

Heterogeneity of Coronary Blood Flow Distribution

Defective tissue oxygen extraction capacity could be due to heterogeneity of coronary blood flow distribution. Herbertson et al. (1995) investigated this question in a porcine endotoxemic model. They measured myocardial blood flow and its distribution, using radiolabeled microspheres. After endotoxin challenge, myocardial oxygen extraction decreased, associated with an increased myocardial blood flow that was heterogeneous. The decrease in oxygen extraction could be explain by the proportional increase in blood flow that was due to a decrease in coronary vascular resistance comparable to that produced by marked pharmacological stimulation. The decrease in oxygen extraction ratio might also have been due to a mismatching of myocardial oxygen delivery to consumption because of the heterogeneity of flow. However, neither myocardial oxygen nor lactate consumption decreased in endotoxemic group, and changes in left ventricular contractility were not correlated with changes in myocardial oxygen extraction. They conclude that the decrease in myocardial oxygen extraction is due to both increased blood flow and mismatching between myocardial oxygen delivery and demand. Impaired myocardial oxygen extraction capacity during sepsis does not cause global myocardial tissue hypoxia.

Role of Leukocytes

As endotoxin administration has been showed to lead to trapping of activated leukocytes in myocardial capillaries, Goddard et al. (1995) tested the hypothesis that leukocytes retained in the coronary circulation could contribute to heterogeneity of myocardial blood flow distribution. They demonstrated, in pigs, that leukocyte were activated following endotoxin infusion, and that activation of leukocytes increased their capillary transit time, as well as their retention in coronary circulation. The potential causes of slowed myocardial capillary transit time of leukocytes following endotoxin exposure include decreased leukocyte deformability and increased leukocyte-endothelial cell adherence. They postulated that leukocytes may contribute to impaired myocardial function in sepsis, just as similar degrees of leukocyte slowing and retention contribute to lung injury in sepsis.

Granton et al. (1997) from the same laboratory elegantly demonstrated that activated leukocytes, retained in the myocardium, in the sepsis-related impaired myocardial contractility. Humoral substances including TNF-α, IL-2, IL-6 released by leukocytes could adversely affect the heart in sepsis. Activated neutrophils may represent a significant source of nitric oxide and neutrophil chemoattractants, and may also produce tissue damage through both oxidative and non-oxidative enzymatic mechanisms. During septic shock, activated neutrophils lead to an increase in vascular permeability and are involved in the development of organ dysfunction. Leukocytes mediate tissue damage and dysfunction in ischemia – reperfusion injury. In dogs, removal of leukocytes from the coronary circulation by filtration reduced myocardial ischemia – reperfusion injury following a period of coronary occlusion (Sheridan et al. 1991). The blockade of coronary endothelial adhesion to neutrophils produced by administrating antibodies to either CD-11b, CD-18, L-selectin or ICAM-1 has been shown to attenuate myocardial ischemia-reperfusion injury and dysfunction (Ma et al. 1991; Ma et al. 1993).

Beneficial Effect of NO Production

The pattern of disordered coronary flow regulation may be due to the release of a putative vasodilator substance such as NO (Kostic et al. 1996). Recent evidence suggests that a massive release of NO, a very potent endogenous vasodilator, causes much of the vascular relaxation and hypotension during sepsis or endotoxemia. Under physiological conditions, NO plays an important role in the regulation of blood pressure and tissue perfusion. In sepsis and endotoxemia, an inducible form of NO synthase, located in vascular smooth muscle, is formed; this process leads to a massive release of NO, resulting in profound vasodilatation. Garcia et al. (1996) showed that NO may produce a basal coronary vasodilator tone and may inhibit endothelin-1-induced coronary vasoconstriction. In the coronary vessels, NO plays a role in the regulation of myocardial blood flow. Avontuur et al. (1995) investigated the role of NO in the hyperdynamic changes of coronary flow in hearts of endotoxin-treated rats. They indicated that these vascular changes are predominantly due to the vasodilatory action of NO. However, inhibition of the NO pathway can result in focal areas of ischemia in endotoxin-treated hearts, suggesting an imbalance of local oxygen supply to demand (Fig. 4).

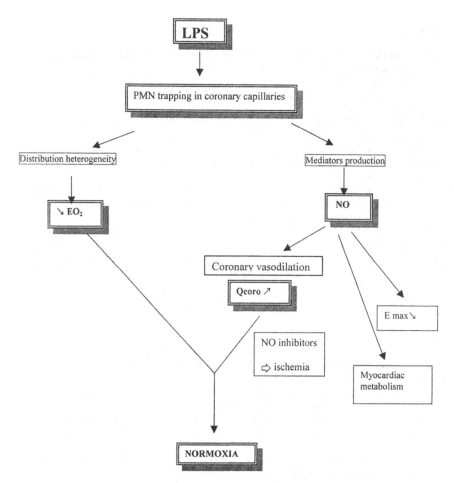

Fig. 4. Schematic representation of the effects of endotoxin (*LPS*) in polymorphonuclear (*PMN*) trapping in coronary capillaries, mediators production, and distribution heterogeneity. Note that the induction of NO synthase in the myocardium during endotoxemia may be a protective mechanism that prevents the development of local ischemia of malperfused cardiac tissue, and that the inhibition of NO synthesis could be counterproductive

Conclusion

Although this has not been systematically tested for all degrees of contractility and ventricular loading conditions, the heart is unique in that, at different levels of oxygen consumption, it operates close to its critical level of oxygen delivery. The sole counter-regulatory mechanism it possesses, in states of unfavorable oxygen delivery or extraction, is tapping its flow reserve.

Sepsis is characterized by a marked coronary vasodilatation with an endotoxin-induced marked heterogeneity of coronary blood flow distribution. Activated leukocytes may play in role in this heterogeneous distribution of blood, as well as myocardial injury.

References

1. Avontuur JAM, Bruining HA, Ince C (1995). Inhibition of nitric oxide synthesis causes myocardial ischemia in endotoxemic rats. Circ Res 76: 418–425
2. Bloos FM, Morisaki HM, Neal AM, Martin CM, Ellis CG, Sibbald WJ (1996). Sepsis depresses the metabolic oxygen reserve of the coronary circulation in mature sheep. Am J Respir Crit Care Med 153: 1577–1584
3. Cunnion RE, Schaer GL, Parker NM, Natanson C, Parillo JE (1986). The coronary circulation in human septic shock. Circulation 73: 637–644
4. Dhainaut JF, Huyghebaert MF, Monsallier JF, et al. (1987). Coronary hemodynamics and myocardial metabolism of lactate, free fatty acids, glucose, and ketones in patients with septic shock. Circulation 75: 522–541
5. Garcia JL, Fernandez N, Garcia-Villalon AL, Monge L, Gomez B, Dieguez G (1996). Coronary vasoconstriction by endothelin-1 in anesthetized goats: role of endothelin receptors, nitric oxide and prostanoids. Eur J Pharmacol 315 (2): 179–186
6. Goddard CM, Allard MF, Hogg JC, Herbertson MJ, Walley KR (1995). Prolonged leukocyte transit time in coronary microcirculation of endotoxemic pigs. Am J Physiol 269: H1389-H1397
7. Granton JT, Goddard CM, Allard MF, van Eeden S, Walley KR (1997). Leukocytes and decreased left-ventricular contractility during endotoxemia in rabbits. Am J Respir Crit Care Med 155: 1977–1983
8. Groeneveld ABJ, van Lambalgen AA, van den Bos GC, Bronsveld W, Nauta JJ, Thijs LG (1991). Maldistribution of heterogeneous coronary blood flow during canine endotoxin shock. Cardiovasc Res 25: 80–88
9. Herbertson MJ, Werner HA, Russel JA, Iversen K, Walley KR (1995). Myocardial oxygen extraction ratio is decreased during endotoxemia in pigs. J Appl Physiol 79: 479–486
10. Kostic MM, Petronijevic MR, Jakovljevic VL (1996). Role of nitric oxide (NO) in the regulation of coronary circulation. Physiol Res 45 (4): 273–278
11. Ma AI, Tsao PS, Lefer A (1991). Antibody to CD-18 exerts endothelial and cardiac protective effects in myocardial ischemia and reperfusion. J Clin Invest 88: 1237–1243
12. Ma XI, Weirich AS, Lefer DJ et al. (1993). Monoclonal antibody to L-selectin attenuates neutrophil accumulation and protects ischemic reperfused cat myocardium. Circulation 88: 649–658
13. Mosher P, Ross J Jr, McFate PA et al. (1964). Control of coronary blood flow by an autoregulatory mechanism. Circ Res 14: 250–259
14. Schremmer B, Dhainaut JF (1990). Regulation of myocardial oxygen delivery. Intensive Care Med 16: S157-S163
15. Sheridan FM, Dauber IM, McMurtry IF, Lesnefsky EJ, Horwitz LD (1991). Role of leukocytes in coronary vascular endothelial injury due to ischemia and reperfusion. Circ Res 69: 1566–1574

16. Suga H, Hisano R, Goto Y, Yamada O, Igarashi Y (1983). Effects of positive inotropic agents on the relation between oxygen consumption and systolic pressure volume aera in canine left ventricle. Circ Res 53: 306–318

Role of Inflammatory Response and Thrombosis in Acute Coronary Syndromes

A. Fernández Ortiz

Introduction

Atherosclerotic involvement of coronary arteries is the underlying process in the majority of ischemic heart diseases. Atherosclerotic lesions may cause stable syndromes of ischemia by means of direct luminal arterial narrowing (*stable lesions*) or unstable or acute ischemic syndromes by inducing intraluminal thrombus formation (*unstable lesions*). Clinical consequences of coronary lesions will depend on the degree and acuteness of blood flow obstruction, the duration of decreased perfusion and the relative myocardial oxygen demand at the time of blood flow obstruction.

Overall, the term "nonsignificant" when applied to atherosclerotic lesions with less than 50% luminal stenosis at coronary angiography may be often misleading. It is now quite evident that a fissure may develop in an atherosclerotic plaque that occupies less than 50% of the diameter of a coronary artery and such mildly stenotic plaque may become a nidus for thrombosis and acute blood flow impairment. Therefore, it is the pathology of coronary atherosclerosis what provides the basis for understanding clinical outcomes of acute coronary syndromes. The unstable lesion that cause infarction are not necessarily severely stenotic, and stenotic lesions are not necessarily unstable. The risk of an acute event, such as unstable angina or acute myocardial infarction, is ultimately determined by how many vulnerable plaques are present. In the present review, we will discuss those determinants for vulnerability of atherosclerotic lesions as well as factors influencing the thrombotic response that inevitably follows rupture of an atherosclerotic plaque.

Vulnerable Plaque Formation

Atherosclerosis Initiation

In the prevalent view, atherosclerosis is considered a healing response of the arterial wall to various injurious stimuli [1]. Chronic injury to the vessel wall in certain parts of the arterial tree may initially lead to endothelial dysfunction. Such dysfunction is characterized by an increased uptake of low density lipoproteins (LDL) and enhanced monocyte recruitment into the vessel wall, both pivotal initiating events for atherosclerosis. Hypercholesterolemia, hyperglycaemia, chemical irritants in tobacco smoke and circulating vasoactive amines are important causative factors in atherogenesis [2–5], however conventional risk factors do not fully explain the diversity of this disease and why interventions have not reduce its incidence as much as epidemiologists have predicted. Interestingly, an infectious hypothesis for atherogenesis, proposed more than 20 years ago [6–8], could fit well into the currently accepted response-to-injury model of atherogenesis. Chronic infections by inducing endothelial dysfunction and by increasing hypercoagulability could contribute to initiate atherosclerotic lesion formation [9]. Specifically, *Chlamydia pneumonie*, an intracellular microorganism, has been shown in case-controlled studies to be associated with coronary artery disease, atherosclerotic carotid disease, and stroke [10, 11]. However, whether *Chlamydia pneumonie* is an innocent bystander or whether it is a causative factor for endothelial damage, hypercoagulability, and macrophage activation, remains uncertain. Large randomized, double-blind, placebo-controlled studies are underway to elucidate the precise value of antibiotic eradication therapy, at least in those patients with atherosclerotic disease and seropositive for infection [12, 13].

Interestingly, despite exposure of different areas of the endothelial surface to the same injurious stimulae concentration, spontaneous atherosclerotic lesions only develop in certain locations. Clearly, there must be local factors that modulate the impact of hypercholesterolemia and other risk factors on the vessel wall, determining the location and possibly the rate of atherosclerosis progression [14, 15]. In fact, atherosclerotic plaques are located more frequently near bifurcations, near trifurcations, and in curvatures of vessels compared with other sites in the arterial tree [16–18]. A recent study using a three dimensional reconstruction technique to calculate shear stress on the endothelium has shown, for the first time in human vessels in vivo, evidence that low shear stress promotes atherosclerotic plaque formation [19]. Experimentally, endothelial cells undergo morphological alterations in response to change in the degree and orientation of shear forces. Whereas elongated endothelial cells are located in regions of high shear stress, polygonal endothelial cells are located in low shear stress regions [20, 21]. These cellular alterations may well also contribute to explain changes in endothelial cell permeability for atherogenic lipoprotein particles.

Atherosclerosis Progression

Lipid accumulation, macrophage formation and cell proliferation constitute the key events in atherosclerosis progression. If excess influx of lipids predominates over its efflux and over the proliferative response, the atherosclerotic process progresses into the most clinically relevant phase of plaque evolution where the so called unstable lipid-rich lesions develop. Such lesions are characterized by a predominance of extracellular lipids occupying a defined region of the intima and separated from the vascular lumen by a fibrous cap. This extracellular accumulation of lipids is known as the lipid core [22]. Characteristically, the lipid core is relatively avascular and hypocellular containing mainly cholesterol monohydrate, cholesterol esters, and phospholipids. Extracellular deposits of cholesterol esters are water insoluble and form an oil-lipid crystalline phase; however, as lesions progresses, additional extracellular accumulation of free cholesterol results in the formation of cholesterol crystals into the lipid core [23]. Extracellular accumulation of lipids appears to be mainly due to rupture of macrophages and to accumulated debris resulting from cell death [22]. Since the macrophage receptor for modified LDL are not regulated [24], excessive intracellular accumulation of lipoproteins may lead to destruction of the cell with subsequent release of oxidized LDL and free radicals into the extracellular space. The lipid core is several orders of magnitude softer that the fibrous cap [25]. This mechanical property is likely to be a critical factor in determining plaque stability. The softer the lipid core, the more stress the overlying fibrous cap must bear and the higher the likelihood of plaque rupture.

Alternatively, if at early stages of atherosclerotic plaque evolution, smooth muscle cell proliferation and extracellular matrix synthesis predominates over macrophage entry and lipid accumulation into the vessel wall, atherosclerotic lesions may grow by means of fibrointimal proliferation giving rise to an advanced sclerotic plaque. Such lesions consist entirely or almost entirely of scar collagen, and lipid may have regressed or it may never have been in the lesion [22, 23]. Lesions that are primarily fibrotic, while they may cause very serious stenosis, are very seldom the site of thrombosis. Factors determining whether a lesion evolves as a primarily fibrotic lesion or as a primarily lipid-rich lesion are actually under intensive investigation. It has been speculated that if the apoptotic cells are mostly cleared by phagocitosis before damage to the plasma membrane causes the cell contents to leak, a fibrotic lesions may develop. On the other hand, if a foam cell become necrotic (either because adjacent macrophages fail to engulf it or because its apoptotic program is defective), there will be a progressive accumulation of lipid in the extracellular space and the lesion may evolve to be an unstable thrombosis-prone type of lesion. Thus, the cell-scavenging function of macrophages may be playing a role both in the initiation of the lesion and in the evolution that determines whether it will be stable or unstable.

Plaque Vulnerability to Rupture

Plaque rupture is a mechanical event that depends on an imbalance between the stress imposed on the plaque cap in systole and the innate strength (resistance to fracture) of the cap tissue. Morphological features that characterize de unstable atheroma include a large necrotic core of lipids and cellular debris an a thin fibrous cap [26]. This plaque configuration is particularly unstable because large mechanical stresses develop in the thinnest portion of the fibrous cap [27, 28]. The soft lipid core is unable to bear the mechanical forces, and excess stresses are thus concentrated in the fibrous cap. Computer modeling analysis of tensile stress across the vessel wall has shown high concentrations of stress at the ends of the caps overlaying an area of lipid pool (the shoulder region), particularly when the lipid pool exceeds ~45% of the vessel wall circumference [25, 28]. In addition, marked oscillations in shear stress, acute change in coronary pressure or tone, and bending and twisting of an artery during each heart contraction could also contribute to plaque rupture.

Moreover, recent observations tell us that other critical factors may also contribute to the ultimate fracture of the fibrous cap. Atheromas with similar geometric features rupture and others do not [29]. A body of consistent evidence supports the view that the extracellular matrix of the fibrous cap is a dynamic, biologically active environment. It is now clear that some degree of ongoing matrix degradation is a highly controlled and essential component of normal tissue homeostasis. There are three major pathways of extracellular matrix degradation: the serine proteases, which include urokinase-type plasminogen activator and plasmin; the cysteine proteases; and the matrix metalloproteinases (MMPs). The fibrous cap matrix may therefore be weakened by enzimatic degradation. Experiments showing an increase in collagen breakdown when monocyte-derived macrophage are incubated with human aortic plaques [30] clearly indicate that macrophages could be responsible for plaque disruption. In addition, atherectomy specimens obtained from patients with unstable coronary syndromes have revealed significantly larger macrophage-rich areas compared with patients with stable angina [31], further supporting that macrophages play a crucial roll in the inflammatory component of the acute coronary syndromes. Activated macrophages may synthesize and secrete MMPs into the extracellular space. Several works have shown increased gene expression and presence of immunoreactive enzymes in the human atheroma [32–34] but, more interestingly, it has been demonstrated by in situ zymography that excess matrix degrading activity is indeed present in the human atheroma, particularly in the shoulder region of the atheroma, were mechanical stresses are highest [35]. Most MMPs are secreted as proenzymes and they must be activated into the extracellular space. Mechanism of in vivo MMP activation is unclear and may involve plasmin, urokinase-type plasminogen activator, membrane-type MMPs, or even autoactivation [36]. Even after MMPs are activated, they may be inhibited. Specific endogenous inhibitors called tissue inhibitors of metalloproteinases (TIMPs) have an amino-terminal domain that binds to available MMP active sites on a 1:1 stoichiometric basis, thereby inhibiting these enzymes [37, 38].

Another fascinating pathological observation is that fibrous cap that have ruptured have not only twice as many macrophages as unruptured fibrous caps but also half as many smooth muscle cells. Therefore, at the same time that inflammation and matrix degradation decrease plaque strength, inadequate numbers of smooth muscle cells may be present to repair the degradation. Recent findings suggest that smooth muscle cells of the atheroma undergo programmed cell death or apoptosis [39, 40]. The precise signals that regulate apoptosis in the atheroma are unknown, as multiple stimuli can provoke this process. Some proteins, including IL-1β-converting enzyme, TNF-α, interferon-γ, or the tumor suppresser p53 sometimes function as apoptosis on signals, while genes such as bcl-2 can function as apoptosis off genes [41, 42]. Lack of sufficient smooth muscle cells to secrete and organize the matrix in response to mechanical stress could render the fibrous cap even more vulnerable to weakening by extracellular matrix degradation.

Markers of Inflammation

Advances in our knowledge of the molecular basis of atherosclerosis make possible the development of molecular markers that can be measured in plasma or serum and used for the identification of individuals at high risk of coronary events. Data from recent clinical trials [43–46] strongly support the position that C-reactive protein (CRP), as a marker of low-level inflammation, indicates increased risk of myocardial infarction and stroke in otherwise healthy individuals. Other acute-phase reactants, such as fibrinogen, factor VIII and plasminogen activator inhibitor-1, have been shown in a wide variety of studies to consistently predict future cardiovascular events [47–50]. Cytokines mediators of inflammation themselves, specifically IL-6, are also risk factors for ischemic heart disease [51]. In addition, it has been also hypothesized that cellular adhesion molecules may provide an indirect molecular marker for pre-clinical atherosclerosis. Two prospective studies have recently shown the first evidence that plasma concentration of at least one cellular adhesion molecule, intercellular adhesion molecule type-1 (ICAM-1), are indeed elevated many years in advance of developing clinical coronary disease [52, 53]. All these findings raise several questions: first, are all of these markers equivalent with respect to risk prediction?, second, is the inflammation that these measures reflect an epiphenomenon of atherosclerotic disease or is it in the cardiovascular event causal pathway?, third, are these markers independent of other estimates of subclinical cardiovascular disease?, and fourth, should anti-inflammatory intervention strategies be considered for those patients at increased risk?. Future investigations will bring some answers to these important questions.

Thrombus Formation

It is likely that many variables determine whether a ruptured plaque proceeds rapidly to an occlusive thrombus with the potential for acute ischemic events or persists at an intermediate stage as a mural non-occlusive clinically silent thrombus. Local factors such as quantity (fissure size), quality of thrombogenic substrate (plaque composition) and rheology of blood flow at the site of plaque rupture, together with systemic factors inducing hypercoagulable or thrombogenic states (chatecolamines, lipoprotein (a), fibrinolytic system) modulate thrombosis at the time of plaque rupture.

Local Thrombogenic Factors

Degree of Plaque Disruption. Experimentally, exposure of subendothelial superficial layers to flowing blood at high shear rate (mimicking a stenosed coronary artery) induces platelet adhesion and aggregation, but the thrombus is labile and may be partially dislodged from the substrate by the flowing blood leaving a small residual mural thrombus [54, 55]. However, exposure of deeper vascular layers to flowing blood produces a dense platelet thrombus that cannot be easily dislodged [54, 55]. As a clinical counterpart, probably when only the surface of a coronary plaque is eroded, the thrombogenic stimulus is relatively limited, resulting in small mural thrombosis with subsequent thrombus organization and asymptomatic growth of the lesion. However a greater degree of plaque damage may be marker of more extensive coronary thrombus formation leading to unstable angina, and an even more complex atherosclerotic plaque rupture may lead to persistent thrombotic coronary occlusion responsible for acute myocardial infarction.

Tissue Substrate. Two retrospective clinical studies suggesting that myocardial infarction developed more frequently from previous nonsevere coronary lesions [56, 57], and a recent angiographic study showing that the atheromatous plaque substrate may be different in Q-wave and non Q-wave myocardial infarction [58] support the idea that plaque composition may be more important than plaque size for developing acute coronary syndromes. Experimentally, the thrombotic response is influenced by the various components of the atherosclerotic plaque exposed following rupture. Exposure of macrophage-rich or collagen-rich matrix, which might be present in superficial plaque erosions or small plaque fissures, is associated with less platelet deposition than that seen after exposure of the lipid-rich core of the plaque [59]. The lipid core is about 6-fold more thrombogenic than the collagen-rich component of the plaque [59] (Fig. 1). Therefore, atheromatous plaques containing lipid-rich "gruel" are not only the most vulnerable plaque to rupture, they are also the most thrombogenic when their content is exposed to flowing blood. Although, the component(s) responsible for such high thrombogenicity found in the lipid-core is unknown, tissue factor protein (derived from disintegrated macrophages?) has been proposed as a key factor initiating the thrombotic response. Tissue factor protein has been identified immunohistochemically in a scattered pattern within the atheromatous core of human plaques [60], tissue factor expression has been more frequently found on macrophages in the coronary plaques of patients with unstable angina [61, 62] and, more importantly, tissue factor has been recently demonstrated as a mediator of the increased thrombogenicity of atheromatous lesions by use of an in situ binding assay for factor VIIa [63]. However, it is likely that others components of the gruel, such as lipids or collagen degradation products, might also contribute to induce platelet aggregation and activation of the coagulation system.

Degree of Stenosis. Acute thrombotic response to plaque disruption depends also in part on the degree of stenosis and sudden geometric changes following the rupture [64]. High shear rates at the site of a significant stenosis will predispose to increased platelet and fibrin(ogen) deposition by forcing both to the periphery where they may be deposited at the site of plaque damage [55, 65, 66]. A small geometric change with only mild stenosis may result in a small mural thrombus, whereas a larger geometric change with severe stenosis may result in a transient or persistent thrombotic occlusion. Furthermore, the disruption of a plaque at the apex of an stenosis may result in a thrombus that is richer in platelets [54, 55] and, therefore, less amenable to fibrinolytic agents than a thrombus formed in a zone distal to the apex [54, 55, 65].

Surface Roughness. Besides degree of stenosis and the nature of the exposed thrombogenic material, fibrous cap disruption produces a rough surface within

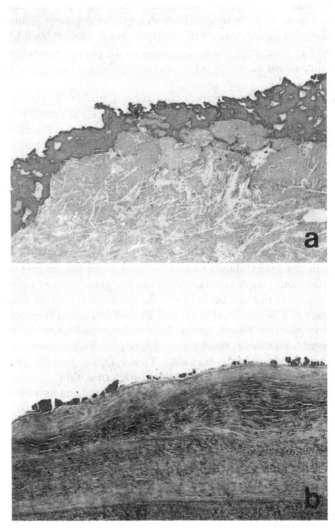

Fig. 1a,b. Relative thrombogenicity of the different components of atherosclerotic plaques. Exposure of the lipid-core with abundant cholesterol crystals (**a**) to flowing blood, in an ex-vivo perfusion system, resulted in a higher thrombus formation than exposure of collagen-rich matrix (**b**) (see [59]). Original magnification ×75

the arterial lumen that further stimulates the development of acute thrombosis. Data derived from ex-vivo perfusion studies on human aortic atherosclerotic plaques have shown that the roughness of the exposed surface, measured by presence of microscopic flaps, dissections, fissures and surface irregularities at the site of plaque rupture, also influences thrombogenicity [59]. As roughness increases, thombogenicity increases probably due to the effect of local flow disturbances on the surface of the ruptured plaque.

Residual Thrombus. After spontaneous lysis, residual mural thrombus predisposes to recurrent thrombotic occlusion [67–69]. Several factors that contribute to rethrombosis have been identified. The residual mural thrombus may encroach into the vessel lumen, resulting in increased stenosis and an increased shear rate, which facilitates the activation and deposition of platelets and fibrin-ogen [55, 65, 70]. After thrombolysis, thrombin bound to fibrin may become exposed to the circulating blood leading to platelet and clotting activation and further thrombosis [71–73]. Clinical studies have also suggested that the enhancement of platelet and thrombin activity by thrombolytic agents themselves may contribute to rethrombosis [74, 75].

Systemic Thrombogenic Factors

Besides local factors, clinical and experimental evidence have suggested that systemic factors inducing a primary hypercoagulable or thrombogenic state may be responsible for formation of a large thrombus after plaque disruption.

High Levels of Catecholamines. Platelet activation and the generation of thrombin may be enhanced by high levels of sympathetic activity [76, 77]. Whereas much of the epinephrine-thrombogenic mechanism may be related to potentiation of other thrombogenic factors, such as serotonin, ADP and thromboxane A_2 [78], the effect of norepinephrin on platelet function is controversial [79, 80]. A recent experimental study has shown opposing effects of plasma epinephrin and norepinephrin on coronary thrombosis [80]. It is likely that activities and conditions such as smoking and mental stress, in which a proportional greater increase is observed in epinephrine, are associated with an elevated risk of thrombosis, whereas during exercise, where plasma norepinephrine tends to be proportionally greater, a diminished risk of thrombosis exists [80].

Cholesterol Levels, Lipoprotein (a), and Other Metabolic States. Hypercholesterolemia has been associated with hypercoagulability and enhanced platelet reactivity manifested at the site of experimentally induced acute vascular damage [81], but mechanisms underlying the effect of high serum cholesterol level on acute thrombus formation remain unclear.

Lp (a) is an important risk factor for ischemic heart disease, particularly in persons with familial hypercholesterolemia or with a family history of premature coronary disease [82]. Apo (a) is a glycoprotein present in Lp (a) that has close structural homology with plasminogen, with both genes being clearly linked on the long arm of chromosome 6 [83]. There is evidence to suggest that the close homology of Lp (a) with plasminogen results in competitive inhibition of the fibrinolytic properties of plasminogen [84], thus predisposing patients to acute thrombotic complications. In a recent angiographic study, patients with rapid progression of coronary artery disease were found to have an increased level of Lp (a) when compared to those without progression, further supporting the role of Lp (a) in atherosclerotic disease [85].

A decrease in HDL-associated Apo A-1 in patients with unstable angina and during the acute phase of myocardial infarction has suggested that HDL may also play a part in preventing intracoronary thrombus formation [86]. In addition to the generally accepted biochemical property of HDL to prevent the accumulation of cholesterol, it has been suggested that HDL stabilizes PGI_2 through a newly discovered function of Apo A-1, which is associated with the surface of HDL particles and identified as PGI_2 stabilizing factor [86].

Other metabolic abnormalities, such as diabetes mellitus, may enhance platelet reactivity and coagulation, perhaps through an increase in plasma von Willebrand factor [87], or through an alteration of the free cholesterol content of platelet membranes secondary to the changes of plasma lipoproteins [88]. Consistent with the enhancement in thrombogenicity, a substantial increase in the incidence of myocardial infarction and microangiopathy has been observed in nonintensively treated diabetics [89, 90]. Other metabolic conditions, such as heterozygous homocystinuria or homocystinemia, are considered to be more atherogenic than thrombogenic risk factors.

Enhanced Platelet and Coagulation Activity, Impaired Fibrinolysis, and High Fibrinogen and Factor VII Levels. The above discussion on the effects of cathecholamines, cholesterol and diabetes on enhancing platelet and coagulation activity and myocardial infarction opens the possibility that activated platelets and coagulation may be thrombogenic risk factors in patients with coronary disease. A recent study suggests that in patients with coronary disease, enhanced thrombin-induced platelet aggregation is a marker for subsequent acute coronary events and disease progression [91]. It is also of interest that patients, long after clinical stabilization of an acute coronary syndrome, exhibit an increased basal levels of thrombin generation as measured by serum fragments 1 and 2, and of thrombin activity as measured by serum fibrinopeptide A, suggesting that such increased activity may serve as a trigger of the primary or recurrent ischemic events [92]. Most important, other hemostatic proteins, specifically fibrinogen and factor VII, have been implicated as major thrombogenic risk factors. Several prospective studies have shown a high plasma fibrinogen concentration to be highly significant independent risk factor for coronary artery disease, specifically associated with myocardial infarction [93]. High levels of factor VII coagulant activity are also associated with an increased risk of coronary events [93]. Both proteins are elevated in relation to age, obesity, hyperlipidemia, diabetes, smoking and emotional stress [94, 95], thus they may also explain partially the effect of other risk factors associated with the disease.

Clinical Consequences of Coronary Plaque Rupture

Not every plaque disruption results in an acute coronary event. In fact, plaque rupture that culminates into an acute coronary syndrome is the "exception rather than the rule" [64, 96]. Postmortem studies have reported that plaque ruptures can be found in 9% of subjects who died of noncardiac causes and in as many as 22% of patients with diabetes or hypertension [97]. Fractured fibrous caps with intense inflammation are also a common finding in the abdominal aorta at necropsy, and asymptomatic carotid plaque rupture may be found in almost one

fifth of elderly persons at autopsy [98]. Plaque rupture with nonocclusive thrombus formation and activation of the inflammatory and reparative processes may
be an important mechanism of asymptomatic plaque growth [99, 100). This
hypothesis has been for years overshadowed by a large body of literature on lipids
and lipoproteins. However, recent angiographic studies have shown unequivocal-
ly that the progression of early atherosclerotic lesions to clinically manifest,
enlarging atherosclerotic plaques, such as those which cause blood flow impairment, is frequently neither lineal nor predictable [56, 57]. While the process of
lipid accumulation, cell proliferation, and extracellular matrix synthesis may be
expected to be linear with time, new high-grade lesions often appear in segments
of arteries that were normal at previous angiographic examination. Moreover,
analysis of the coronary tree in patients who died of ischemic heart disease has
shown a morphological appearance consistent with previously healed fissures at
different stages of thrombosis and thrombus organization [101], and fibrinogen
and fibrin concentration in cholesterol-rich advanced plaques have been found to
be 10 times higher than in normal vessels [102]. Therefore, it may well be that the
healing organization process of intraplaque thrombi contributes to subclinical
progression of the lesions through interactions between thrombotic elements and
vascular cells. Besides platelets (1,103), thrombin has been shown to be a potent
mitogen for mesenchimal derived cells and it is chemotactic for monocytes [104,
105], and fibrinogen and its degradation products may also contribute to lesion
progression by their ability to stimulate vascular cell proliferation [106]. Thus,
thrombus formation in an artery may not only lead to occlusion of the vessel
[107], but also contribute to the development of the atheromatous lesion itself.

However, although most ruptured plaques could be resealed by a small mural
thrombus, occasionally large thrombi can impair coronary blood flow leading to
acute syndromes of myocardial ischemia. The amount and duration of intracoronary thrombus play a major pathophysiologic role in clinical presentation [64,
108, 109). In general, acute myocardial infarction is associated with larger and
more persistent thrombus than is unstable angina. In unstable angina, a relatively small fissuring or disruption of the plaque may lead to an acute change in
plaque structure and a reduction in coronary blood flow, resulting in exacerba-
tion of angina. Transient episodes of thrombotic vessel occlusion at the site of
plaque rupture may occur, leading to angina at rest. This thrombus is usually
labile and results in temporary vascular occlusion, perhaps lasting only
10–20 min. In non-Q wave infarction, more severe plaque damage would result in
more persistent thrombotic occlusion, perhaps lasting up to 1 h. About one fourth
of patients with non-Q wave infarction may have an infarct-related vessel occluded for more than 1 h, but the distal myocardial territory is usually supplied by collaterals. Resolution of vasospasm may be also pathogenically important in non-Q
wave infarction. In Q wave infarction, larger plaque fissures may result in the formation of a large, fixed and persistent thrombus. This leads to an abrupt cessation
of myocardial perfusion for more than 1 h resulting in transmural necrosis of the
involved myocardium. The coronary lesion responsible for the infarction is frequently only mildly to moderately stenotic, which supports that plaque rupture
with superimposed thrombus rather than the severity of the lesion is the primary determinant of acute occlusion. In summary, the natural history of acute coro-

nary syndromes probably mirrors that of the underlying plaque rupture and thrombus formation. Stabilization would correspond to resealing of a rupture, accentuation of symptoms to development of labile thrombosis, non-Q wave infarction to development of transient occlusion, and transmural Q-wave infarction to establishment of a persistent occlusive thrombus.

References

1. Ross R: The pathogenesis of atherosclerosis: a perspective for the 1990s. Nature 1993, 362:801–809
2. Seiler C, Hess OM, Buechi M, Suter TM, Krayenbuehl HP. Influence of serum cholesterol and other coronary risk factors on vasomotion of angiographically normal coronary arteries. Circulation 1993, 88:2139–2148
3. Vita JA, Treasure CB, Nabel EG, et al: Coronary vasomotor response to acetylcholine relates to risk factors for coronary artery disease. Circulation 1990, 81:491–497
4. Feener EP, King GL. Vascular dysfunction in diabetes mellitus. Lancet 1997, 350 (suppl I): 9–13
5. Tell GS, Polak JF, Ward BJ, Kittner SJ, Savage PJ, Robbins J. Relation of smoking with carotid arterial wall thickness and stenosis in older adults: The Cardiovascular Healt Study. Circulation 1994, 90:2905–2908
6. Fabricant CG, Knook L, Gillespie JH. Virus-induced cholesterol crystals. Science 1973 1973, 181:566–567
7. Fabricant CG, Fabricant J, Litrenta MM, Minick CR. Virus-induced atherosclerosis. J Exp Med 1978, 148:335–340
8. Hajjar DP. Viral pathogenesis of atherosclerosis. Am J Pathol 1991, 139:1195–1211
9. Vallance P, Collier J, Bhagat K. Infection, inflammation and infarction: does acute endothelial dysfunction provide a link?. Lancet 1997, 349:1391–1392
10. Cook PJ, Lip GYH. Chlamydia pneumoniae and atherosclerotic vascular disease. Q J Med 1996, 89:727–735
11. Gupta S, Camm AJ. Chlamydia pneumoniae and coronary heart disease. BMJ 1997, 514:1778–1779
12. Lip GYH, Beevers DG. Can we treat coronary artery disease with antibiotics?. Lancet 1997, 350:378–379
13. Libby P, Egan D, Skarlatos S. Roles of infectious agents in atherosclerosis and restenosis. An assessment of the evidence and need for future research. Circulation 1997, 96:4095–4103
14. Gibson CM, Diaz L, Kandarpa K, et al: Relation of vessel wall shear stress to atherosclerosis progression in human coronary arteries. Atherosc Thromb 1993, 13:310–315
15. Asakura T, Karino T: Flow patterns and spatial distribution of atherosclerotic lesions in human coronary arteries. Circ Res 1990, 66:1045–1066
16. Tjotta E. The distribution of atheromatosis in the coronary arteries. J Atheroscler Res 1963; 3: 253–261
17. Sakata N, Takebayashi S. Localization of atherosclerotic lesion in tha curving sites of human internal carotid arteries. Biorheology 1988, 25:567–578
18. Smedby O, Johanson J, Molgaard J, Osen JA, Waldius G, Erikson U. Predilection of atherosclerosis for the inner curvature in femoral artery. Arteriorscler Tromb Vasc Biol 1995, 15:912–917
19. Krams R, Wentzel JJ, Oomen JAF, Schuurbiers JCH, de Feyter PJ, Serruys PW, Slager CJ. Evaluation of endothelial shear stress and 3D geometry as factors determining the development of atherosclerosis and remodeling in human coronary arteries in vivo. Arterioscler Thromb Vasc Biol 1997, 17:2061–2065
20. Levesque MJ, Liepsch D, Moravec S, Nerem RM. Correlation of endothelial cell shape and wall shear stress in a stenosed dog aorta. Arteriosclerosis 1986, 6:220–229

21. Reidy MA, Bowyer D: Scanning electron microscopy of arteries: the morphology of aortic endothelium in hemodynamically stressed areas associated with branches. Atherosclerosis 1977; 26: 181–194

22. A definition of advances types of atherosclerotic lesions and a historical classification of atherosclerosis: A report from the Committe of Vascular Lesions of the Council of Arteriosclerosis, American Heart Association. Stary HC, Chandler AB, Dinsmore RE, Fuster V, Glagov S, Insull W Jr, Rosenfeld ME, Schawrtz CJ, Wagner WD, Wissler RW. Circulation 1995, 92:1355–1374

23. Stary HC: Composition and classification of human atherosclerotic lesions. Virchows Archiv A Pathol Anat 1992, 421:277–290

24. Goldstein JL, Ho YK, Basu SK, Brown MS. Binding site on macrophages that mediates uptake and degradation of acetylated low density lipoprotein, producing massive cholesterol deposition. Proc Natl Acad Sci USA 1979, 76:333–337

25. Loree HM, Tobias BJ, Gibson LJ, Kamm RD, Small DM, Lee RT. Mechanical properties of model atherosclerotic lesion lipid pools. Arterioscler Thromb 1994, 14:230–234

26. Kragel AH, Reddy SG, Wittes JT, Roberts WC. Morphometric analysis of the composition of atherosclerotic plaques in the four major epicardial coronaries in acute myocardial infarction and sudden coronary death. Circulation 1989, 80:1747–1756

27. MacIsaac AI, Thomas JD, Topol EJ: Toward the quiescent coronary plaque. J Am Coll Cardiol 1993, 22:1228–1241

28. Richardson RD, Davies MJ, Born GVR: Influence of plaque configuration and stress distribution on fissuring of coronary atherosclerotic plaques. Lancet 1989, 2:941–944

29. Cheng GC, Loree HM, Kamm RD, Fishbein MC, Lee RT. Distribution of circumferential stress in ruptured and stable atherosclerotic lesions. A structural analysis with histopathological correlation. Circulation 1993, 87:1179–1187

30. Shah PK, Falk E, Badimon JJ, Fernandez-Ortiz A, Mailhac A, Villareal-Levy G, Fallon JT, Regnstrom J, Fuster V. Human monocyte-derived macrophages induce collagen breakdown in fibrous caps of atherosclerotic plaques: potential role of matrix-degrading metalloproteinases and implications for plaque ruprure. Circulation 1995, 92:1565–1569

31. Moreno P, Falk E, Palacios IF, Newell JB, Fuster V, Fallon JT. Macrophage infiltration in acute coronary syndromes: implications for plaque rupture. Circulation 1994, 90:775–778

32. Henney AM, Wakeley PR, Davies MJ, Foster K, Hembry R, Murphy G, Humpries SE. Location of stromelysin gene in atherosclerotic plaques using in situ hybridization. Proc Natl Acad Sci USA 1991, 88:8154–8158

33. Nikkari ST, O'Brien KD, Ferguson M, Hatsukami T, Welgus HG, Alpers CE, Clowes AW. Interstitial collagenase (mmp-1) expression in human carotid atherosclerosis.Circulation1995, 92:1393–8

34. Brown DL, Hibbs MS, Kearney M, Loushin C, Isner JM. Identification of 92-kd gelatinase in human coronary atherosclerotic lesions: association of active enzyme synthesis with unstable angina. Circulation 1995, 91:2125–2131

35. Galis ZS, Sukhova GK, Libby P. Microscopic localization of active proteases by in situ zymography: detection of matrix metalloproteinase activity in vascular tissue. Methodol Commun 1995, 9:974–980

36. Werb Z, Mainardi CL, Vater CA, Harris EDJ. Endogenous activation of latent collagenase by reunathoid sinovial cells:evidence for a role of plasminogen activator. N Engl J Med 1997, 296:1017–23

37. Dollery CM, McEwan JR, Henney AM. Matrix metalloproteinases and cardiovascular disease. Cir Res 1995, 77:863–868

38. DeClerk YA, Darville MI, Eeckhout Y, Rousseau GG. Characterization of the promoter on the gene encoding human tissue inhibitor of metalloproteinases-2 (TIMP-2). Gene 1994, 139:185–191

39. Geng Y, Wu Q, Muszynski M, Hansson GK, Libby P. Apoptosis of vascular smooth muscle cells induced by in vivo stimulation with interferon-g, tumor necrosis factor-a, and interleukin-1b. Arterioscler Thromb Vasc Biol 1996, 16:19–27

40. Bennett MR, Evan GI, Schwartz SM. Apoptosis of human vascular smooth muscle cells derived from normal vessels and coronary atherosclerotic plaques. J Clin Invest 1995, 95:2266–2274
41. Geng Y, Libby P. Evidence for apoptosis in advanced human atheroma: colocalization with interleukin-1b-converting enzyme. Am J Pathophysiol 1995, 147:251–266
42. Bennett MR, Evan GI, Schwartz SM. Apoptosis of rat vascular smooth muscel cells is regulated by p53-dependent and -independent pathways. Circ Res 1995, 77:266–273
43. Kuller L, Tracy R, Shaten J, Meilahn E, for the MRFIT Research Group. Relatioship of C-reactive protein and coronary heart disease in the MRFIT nested case-control study. Am J Epidemiol 1996, 144:537–547
44. Ridker P, Cushman M, Stampfer M, Tracy R, Hennekens C. Inflammation, aspirin, and the risk of cardiovascular disease in apparently healthy men. N Eng J Med 1997, 336:973–979
45. Koening W, Froehlich M, Sund M, Doering A, Fischer H, Loewel H, Hutchinson W, Pepys M. C-reactive protein (CRP) predicts risk of coronary heart disease (CHD) in healthy middle-aged men: results from the MONICA-Augsburg cohort study, 1984/85–1992. Circulation 1997, 96 (suppl I):I-99. Abstract
46. Tracy R, Lemaitre R, Psaty B, Ives D, Evans R, Cushman M, Meilahn E, Kuller L. Relationship of C-reactive protein to risk of cardiovascular disease in the elderly: results from the Cardiovascular Health Study and the Rural Health Promotion Orojet. Arterioscler Thromb Vasc Biol 1997, 17:1121–1127
47. Ernst E, Resch K. Fibrinogen as cardiovascular a cardiovascular risk factor: a meta-analysis and review of the literature. Ann Intern Med 1993, 118:956–963
48. Folsom A, Wu K, Rosamond W, Sharrett A, Chambless L. Hemostatic factors and incidence of coronary heart disease in the Atherosclerosis Risk in Communities (ARIC) study. Circulation 1996, 93:662. Abstract
49. Tracy R, Arnold A, Ettinger W, Freid L, Meilahn E, Savage P. Coagulation factor VIII is associated with incident cardiovascular disease and death in the elderly: the Cardiovascular Health Study. Circulation 1996, 94 (supp I):I-457. Abstract
50. Hamsten A, de Faire U, Walldius G, Dahlen G, Szamosi A, Landou C, Blomback M, Wiman B. Plasminogen activator inhibitor in plasma: risk factor for recurrent myocardial infarction. Lancet 1987, 2:3–9
51. Biasucci L, Vitelli A, Liuzzo G, Altamura S, Caligiuri G, Monaco C, Rebuzzi A, Ciliberto G, Maseri A. Elevated levels of interleukin-6 in unstable angina. Circulation 1996, 94:874–877
52. Ridker PM, Hennekens CH, Roitman-Johnson B, Stampfer MJ, Allen J. Plasma concentration of soluble intercellular adhesion molecule 1 and risk of future myocardial infarction in apparently healthy men. Lancet 1998, 351:88–92
53. Hwang S-J, Ballantyne CM, Sharrett AR, et al. Circulating adhesion molecules VCAM-1, ICAM-1, and E-selectin in carotid atherosclerosis and incident coronary heart disease cases. The Atherosclerosis Risk in Communities (ARIC) Study. Circulation 1997, 96:4219–25
54. Badimon L, Badimon JJ, Turitto VT, Vallabhajosula S, Fuster V. Platelet thrombus formation on collagen type I: a model of deep vessel injury: influence of blood rheology, von Willebrand factor, and blood coagulation. Circulation 1988, 78:1431–1442
55. Badimon L, Badimon JJ: Mechanism of arterial thrombosis in nonparallel streamlines: platelet thrombi grow at the apex of stenotic severiiy injured vessel wall: experimental study in the pig model. J Clin Invest 1898, 84:1134–1144
56. Ambrose JA, Tannenbaum MA, Alexopolous D, Hjemdahl-Monsen CE, Leavy J, Weiss M, Borrico S, Gorlin R, Fuster V. Angiographic progression of coronary artery disease and the development of myocardial infarction. J Am Coll Cardiol 1988, 12:56–62
57. Little WC, Constantinescu M, Applequte RJ, Kutcher MA, Burrows MT, Kahl FR, Sontamore WP. Can coronary angiography predict the site of subsequent myocardial infarction in patients with mild-to-moderate coronary artery disease? Circulation 1988, 76:1157–1166
58. Dacanay S, Kennedy HL, Uretz E, Parrillo JE, Klein LW. Morphological and quantitative angiographic analyses of progression of coronary stenoses. A comparison of Q-wave and non-Q-wave myocardial infarction. Circulation 1994, 90:1739–1746

59. Fernández-Ortiz A, Badimon JJ, Falk E, Fuster V, Meyer B, Mailhac A, Weng D, Shah PK, Badimon L. Characterization of the relative thrombogenicity of atherosclerotic plaque components: Implications for consequences of plaque rupture. J Am Coll Cardiol 1994, 23:1562–1569

60. Wilcox JN, Smith KM, Schwartz SM, Gordon D. Localization of tissue factor in normal vessel wall and in the atherosclerotic plaque. Proc Natl Acad Sci USA 1989, 86:2839–2843

61. Moreno PR, Bernardi VH, Lopez-Cuellar J, Murcia AM, Palacios IF, Gold HK, Mehran R, Sharma SK, Nemerson Y, Fuster V, Fallon JT. Macrophages, smooth muscle cells, and tissue factor in unstable angina. Implications for cell-mediated thrombogenicity in acute coronary syndromes. Circulation 1996, 94:3090–3097

62. Kaikita K, Ogawa H, Yasue H, Takeya M, Takahashi K, Saito T, Hayasaki K, Horiuchi K, Takizawa A, Kamikubo Y, Nakamura S. Tissue factor expresion on macrophages in coronary plaques in patients with unstable angina. Arterioscler Thromb Vasc Biol 1997, 17: 2232–2237

63. Toschi V, Gallo R, Lettino M, Fallon JT, Gertz SD, Fernandez-Ortiz A, Chesebro JH, Badimon L, Nemerson Y, Fuster V, Badimon JJ. Tissue factor modulates the thrombogenicity of human atherosclerotic plaques. Circulation 1997. 95:594–599

64. Fuster V: Lewis A Conner Memorial Lecture. Mechanisms leading to myocardial infarction: Insights from studies of vascular biology. Circulation 1994, 90:2126–2146

65. Mailhac A, Badimon JJ, Fallon JT, Fernandez-Ortiz A, Meyer B, Chesebro JH, Fuster V, Badimon L. Effect of an eccentric severe stenosis on fibri(ogen) deposition on severely damaged vessel wall in arterial thrombosis. Relative contribution of fibri(ogen) and platelets. Circulation 1994, 90:988–996

66. Turitto VT, Baungartner HR: Platelet interaction with subendothelium in flowing rabbit blood: effect of blood shear rate. Microvasc Res 1979, 17:38–54

67. Davies SW, Marchart B, Lyons JP, Timmis AD. Irregular coronary lesion morphology after thrombosis predicts early clinical instability. J Am Coll Cardiol 1991, 18:669–674

68. Hackett D, Davie G, Ghierchia S, Maseri A. Intermittent coronary occlusion in acute myocardial infarction: value of combined thrombolytic and vasodilatory therapy. N Eng J Med 1987, 317:1055–9

69. Ohman EM, Topol EJ, Califf RM, et al: An analysis of the cause of early mortality after administration of thrombolytic therapy. Cor Art Dis 1993, 4:957–964

70. Lassila R, Badimon JJ, Vallabhajosula S, Badimon L. Dynamic monitoring of platelet deposition on severely damaged vessel wall in flowing blood: effect of different stenosis on thrombus growth. Arterioclerosis 1990, 10:306–315

71. Meyer BJ, Badimon JJ, Mailhac A, Fernandez-Ortiz A, Chesebro JH, Fuster V, Badimon L. Inhibition of growth of thrombus on fresh mural thrombus. Targeting optimal therapy. Circulation 1994, 90:2432–1438

72. Fitzgerald DJ, Fitzgerald GA: Role of thrombin and thromboxane A_2 in reocclusion following coronary thrombolysis with tissue-type plasminogen activator. Proc Nat Acad Sci USA1989, 86:7585–9

73. Weitz JI, Hudoba M, Massel D, Maragonore J, Hirsh J. Clot bound thrombin is protected from inhibition by heparin-antithrombin III but is susceptible to inactivation by antithrombin III-independent inhibitors. J Clin Invest 1990, 86:385–391

74. Eisenberg PR, Sherman LA, Jaffe AS: Paradoxic elevation of fibrinopeptide A after streptokinase: evidence for continued thrombosis despite intense fibrinolysis. J Am Coll Cardiol 1987, 10:527–529

75. Owen J, Friedman KD, Grossman BA, Wilkins C, Berke AD, Powers ER. Thrombolytic therapy with tissue plasminogen activator or streptokinase induces transient thrombin activity. Blood 1988, 72:616–620

76. Badimon L, Lassila R, Badimon J, et al: An acute surge of epinephrine stimulates platelet deposition to severely damaged vascular wall (Abstract). J Am Coll Cardiol 15:181 A, 1990

77. Kimura S, Nishinaga M, Ozawa T, Shimada K. Thrombin generation as an acute effect of cigarette smoking. Am Heart J 1994, 128:7–11

78. Yao SK, Ober JC, McNatt J, Benedict C, Rosolowsky M, Anderson HV, Cui C, Maffrand JP, Campbell W, Buja LM, Willerson JT. ADP plays an important role in mediating platelets aggregation and cyclic flow variations in vivo in stenosed and endothelium-injured canine coronary arteries. Circ Res 1992, 70:39–48

79. Larson PT, Wallen NH, Hjemdahl P: Norepinephrine-induced platelet activation in vivo is only partly counteracted by aspirin. Circulation 1994, 89:1951–1957

80. Lin H, Young DB: Opposing effects of plasma epinephrin and norepinephrin on coronary thrombosis in vivo. Circulation 1995, 91:1135–1142

81. Badimon JJ, Badimon L, Turitto VT, Fuster V. Platelet deposition at high shear rates is enhanced by high plasma cholesterol levels: in vivo study in a rabitt model. Arterioscler Thromb 1991, 11:395–402

82. Rader DJ, Hoeg JM, Brewer HB Jr: Quantitation of plasma apolipoproteins in the primary and secondary prevention of coronary artery disease. Ann Intern Med 1994, 120:1012–1025

83. Frank SL, Klisak I, Sparkes RS, et al: The apoprotein (a) gene resides on human chromosome 6q26–27 in close proximity to the homologous gene for plasminogen. Hum Genet 1988, 79:352–356

84. Loscalzo J: Lipoprotein (a): a unique risk factor for athero-thrombotic disease. Arteriosclerosis 1990, 10:672–679

85. Terres W, Tatsis E, Pfalzer B, Beil U, Beisiegel H, Hamm CW. Rapid angiographic progression of coronary artery disease in patients with elevated lipoprotein (a). Circulation 1995, 91:948–951

86. Kawai C: Pathogenesis of acute myocardial infarction. Novel regulatory systems of bioactive substances in the vessel wall. Circulation 1994, 90:1033–1043

87. Bensoussan D, Levy-Toledano S, Passa P, Caen J, Caniver J. Platelet hyperaggregation and increased plasma level of von Willebrand factor in diabetics with retinopathy. Diabetologgia 1975, 11:307–312

88. Schwartz CJ, Kelley JL, Valente AJ, Cayatte AJ, Sprague EA, Rozek MM. Pathogenesis of the atherosclerotic lesion: implication for diabetes mellitus. Diabetes Care 1992, 15:1156–1167

89. Jacoby RM, Nesto RW: Acute myocardial infarction in the diabetic patient: pathophysiology, clinical course and prognosis. J Am Coll Cardiol. 1992, 20:736–744

90. The diabetes control and complications trial research group. The effect of intensive treatment of diabetes on the development and progression of long-term complications in insulin-dependent diabetes mellitus. N Eng J Med 1993, 329:977–986

91. Lamb JYT, Latour JG, Lesperance J, Waters D. Platelet aggregation, coronary artery disease progression and future coronary events. Am J Cardiol 1994, 73:333–338

92. Merlini A, Bauer KA, Oltrona L, Ardissino D, Cattaneo M, Belli C, Mannucci PM, Rosenberg RD. Persistent activation of coagulation mechanism in unstable angina and myocardial infarction. Circulation 1994, 90:61–68

93. Meade TW, North WRS, Chakrabarti R, et al: Haemostatic function and cardiovascular death: early results of a prospective study. Lancet 1980, 1:1050–1054

94. McGill DA, Ardlie NG: The relationship between blood fibrinogen level and coronary artery disease. Cor Art Dis 1990, 1:557–566

95. Rosengren A, Wilhelmsen L, Wellin L, Tsipogianni A, Teger-Nilsson AC, Wedel H. Social influences and cardiovascular risk factor as determinat of plasma fibrinogen concentration in a general population sample of middle age men. BMJ 1990, 330:634–638

96. Libby P. Molecular bases of the acute coronary syndromes. Circulation 1995, 91:2844–2850

97. Davies MJ, Bland JM, Hangartner JRW, Angelini A, Thomas AC. Factors influencing the presence or absence of acute coronary artery thrombi in sudden ischemic death. Eur Heart J 1989, 10:203–208

98. Swindland A, Torvik A. Atherosclerotic carotid disease in asymptomatic individuals: a hystological study of 53 cases. Acta Neurol Scand 1988, 9:202–212

99. von Rokitansky C: A Manual of Pathological Anatomy (Day GE, trans.). London, UK: Sydenham Society 1852 (vol 4):261–273

100. Smith EB, Keen GA, Grant A, Stirk Ch. Fate of fibrinogen in human arterial intima. Arteriosclerosis 1990, 10:263–275
101. Davies MJ, Thomas AC. Plaque fissuring: the cause of acute myocardial infarction, sudden ischemic death and crescendo angina. Br Heart J 1985, 53:363–373
102. Smith E: Fibrinogen, fibrin and fibrin degradation products in relation to atherosclerosis. Clin Haematol 1986, 15:355–358
103. Ferns GAA, Raine EW, Sprugel KH, Motani AS, Reidy MA, Ross R. Inhibition of neointimal smooth muscle accumulation after angioplasty by an antibody to PDGF. Science 1991, 253:1129–1132
104. Berk BC, Taubman MB, Griendling KK, et al: Thrombin stimulated events in cultured vascular smooth muscle cells. Biochem J 1991, 265:17334–17340
105. Jones A, Ceczy CL: Thrombin and factor Xa enhance the production of interleukin-1. Immunology 1990, 71:236–241
106. Naito M, Hayashi T, Kuzuya M, et al: Effects of fibrinogen and fibrin on the migration of vascular smooth muscle cells in vitro. Artherosclerosis 1990, 83:9–14
107. Davies MJ, Thomas A: Thrombosis and acute coronary artery lesions in sudden cardiac ischemic death. N Eng J Med 1984, 310:1137–140
108. Fuster V, Badimon L, Badimon JJ, Chesebro JH. The pathogenesis of coronary artery disease and the acute coronary syndromes (part I). N Eng J Med 1992, 326:242–250
109. Fuster V, Badimon L, Badimon JJ, Chesebro JH. The pathogenesis of coronary artery disease and the acute coronary syndromes (part II). N Eng J Med 1992, 326:310–318

Basic Aspects of Fibrinolysis and Thrombolysis

H.R. Lijnen and D. Collen

Introduction

The hypothesis underlying thrombolytic therapy of thromboembolic disease is that early and sustained recanalization prevents cell death, reduces infarct size, preserves organ function, and reduces early and late mortality. Thrombolysis consists of the pharmacological dissolution of the blood clot, by intravenous infusion of plasminogen activators that activate the fibrinolytic system (Fig. 1). The fibrinolytic system includes a proenzyme, plasminogen, which is converted by plasminogen activators to the active enzyme plasmin, which in turn digests fibrin to soluble degradation products. Inhibition of the fibrinolytic system occurs by plasminogen activator inhibitors (mainly plasminogen activator inhibitor-1, PAI-1) and by plasmin inhibitors (mainly α_2-antiplasmin) [1]. Thrombolytic agents that are either approved or under clinical investigation in patients with acute myocardial infarction include streptokinase, recombinant tissue-type plasminogen activator (rt-PA or alteplase), rt-PA derivatives such as reteplase and TNK-rtPA,

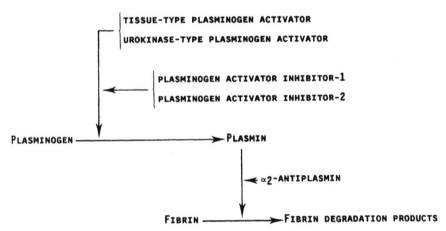

Fig. 1. Schematic representation of the fibrinolytic system. The proenzyme plasminogen is activated to the active enzyme plasmin by tissue-type or urokinase-type plasminogen activator. Plasmin degrades fibrin into soluble fibrin degradation products. Inhibition of the fibrinolytic system may occur at the level of the plasminogen activators, by plasminogen activator inhibitors, or at the level of plasmin, mainly by α_2-antiplasmin

anisoylated plasminogen-streptokinase activator complex (APSAC or anistreplase), two-chain urokinase-type plasminogen activator (tcu-PA or urokinase), recombinant single-chain u-PA (scu-PA, pro-u-PA or prourokinase), and recombinant staphylokinase and derivatives [2].

Although all thrombolytic agents act by converting plasminogen to plasmin, which dissolves the fibrin of blood clots, they are not all equal. Indeed, physiological fibrinolysis is regulated by specific molecular interactions between its main components tissue-type plasminogen activator (t-PA), plasminogen and fibrin. As a result, plasminogen is preferentially activated at the fibrin surface, where generated plasmin is protected from rapid inhibition by α_2-antiplasmin and thus may efficiently degrade the clot [3]. Thus fibrin-selective agents (rt-PA and derivatives, staphylokinase and derivatives and to a lesser extent scu-PA) which digest the clot in the absence of systemic plasminogen activation are distinguished from non fibrin-selective agents (streptokinase, tcu-PA and APSAC) which activate systemic and fibrin-bound plasminogen relatively indiscriminately (Fig. 2). Non fibrin-selective agents are less efficient for clot dissolution and cause a systemic generation of plasmin, depletion of α_2-antiplasmin and degradation of coagulation factors, which however protects against reocclusion of the infarct-related artery [1]. In this contribution, we will review the basic mechanisms regulating fibrinolysis and thrombolysis, mainly with fibrin-specific thrombolytic agents.

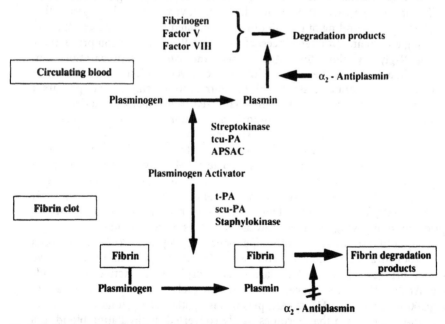

Fig. 2. Molecular interactions determining the fibrin-specificity of plasminogen activators. Non-fibrin-specific plasminogen activators (streptokinase, tcu-PA, APSAC) activate both plasminogen in the fluid phase and fibrin-associated plasminogen. Fibrin-specific plasminogen activators (t-PA, scu-PA, staphylokinase and to a lesser extent reteplase) preferentially activate fibrin-associated plasminogen

Protein Structure of the Main Components of the Fibrinolytic System

Human plasminogen is a 92 kDa single-chain glycoprotein, consisting of 791 amino acids; it contains 24 disulfide bridges and 5 homologous kringles [4]. Native plasminogen has NH_2-terminal glutamic acid ("Glu-plasminogen") but is easily converted by limited plasmic digestion to modified forms with NH_2-terminal lysine, valine, or methionine, commonly designated "Lys-plasminogen". The plasminogen kringles contain lysine binding sites that mediate the specific binding of plasminogen to fibrin and the interaction of plasmin with α_2-antiplasmin; they play a crucial role in the regulation of fibrinolysis [5].

Tissue-type plasminogen activator (t-PA) is a 70 kDa serine proteinase, originally isolated as a single polypeptide chain of 527 amino acids [6]. It was subsequently shown that native t-PA contains an NH_2-terminal extension of three amino acids (Gly-Ala-Arg-). t-PA is converted by plasmin to a two chain form by hydrolysis of the Arg^{275}-Ile^{276} peptide bond. The NH_2-terminal region is composed of several domains with homologies to other proteins: a finger domain comprising residues 4–50, a growth factor domain comprising residues 50–87 and two kringles comprising residues 87–176 and 176–262. The region constituted by residues 276–527 represents the serine proteinase part with the catalytic site, composed of His^{322}, Asp^{371}, and Ser^{478} [6]. These distinct domains in t-PA are involved in several functions of the enzyme, including its binding to fibrin, fibrin-specific plasminogen activation, rapid clearance in vivo and binding to endothelial cell receptors. Binding of t-PA to fibrin is mediated via the finger and the second kringle domains [for references, cf 7]. The t-PA molecule comprises three potential N-glycosylation sites, at Asn^{117}, Asn^{184} and Asn^{448}. t-PA preparations usually contain a mixture of variant I (with all three glycosylation sites) and variant II (lacking carbohydrate at Asn^{184}) [6]. In contrast to the single-chain precursor form of most serine proteinases, single-chain t-PA is enzymatically active.

Single-chain urokinase-type plasminogen activator (scu-PA) is a 54 kDa glycoprotein containing 411 amino acids [8]. Upon proteolytic cleavage of the Lys^{158}-Ile^{159} peptide bond, the molecule is converted to a two-chain derivative (tcu-PA). The catalytic triad is located in the COOH-terminal polypeptide chain and is composed of Asp^{255}, His^{204} and Ser^{356}. The NH_2-terminal chain contains an epidermal growth factor domain (residues 5–49) and one kringle domain. A low Mr tcu-PA (33 kDa) can be generated with plasmin by hydrolysis of the Lys^{135}-Lys^{136} peptide bond following previous cleavage of the Lys^{158}-Ile^{159} bond.

Alpha$_2$-antiplasmin is a 70 kDa single-chain glycoprotein containing about 13% carbohydrate. The molecule consists of 464 amino acids and contains two disulfide bridges [9, 10]. α_2-Antiplasmin is a serpin with reactive site peptide bond Arg^{376}-Met^{377}. Its concentration in normal human plasma is about 7 mg/100 ml (about 1 µM). α_2-Antiplasmin is synthesized primarily in a plasminogen-binding form that becomes partly converted in circulating blood to a non-plasminogen-binding form (about 30% of the total), that lacks a 26-residue peptide from the COOH-terminal end [11]. The inhibitor is cross-linked to the fibrin α chain when blood is clotted in the presence of calcium ions and activated coagulation factor XIII; Gln^{14} is involved in this cross-linking [12].

Plasminogen activator inhibitor-1 (PAI-1) is a 52 kDa single-chain glycoprotein consisting of 379 amino acids; it is a serpin with reactive site peptide bond Arg[346]-Met[347] [13] PAI-1 is stabilized by binding to S-protein or vitronectin [14]; the PAI-1 binding site on vitronectin was mapped to the region comprising residues Lys[348] to Arg[370] [15].

Mechanisms Involved in Inhibition of the Fibrinolytic System

The fibrinolytic system is regulated by controled activation and inhibition. Activation of plasminogen by t-PA is enhanced in the presence of fibrin or at the endothelial cell surface. Inhibition of fibrinolysis occurs at the level of plasminogen activation or at the level of plasmin. Fibrinolysis may also be regulated as a result of increased or decreased synthesis and/or secretion of t-PA and of PAI-1, primarily from the vessel wall.

Inhibition of Plasmin by α_2-Antiplasmin

α_2-Antiplasmin forms an inactive 1:1 stoichiometric complex with plasmin. The inhibition of plasmin (P) by α_2-antiplasmin (A) can be represented by two consecutive reactions: a fast, second order reaction producing a reversible inactive complex (PA), which is followed by a slower first-order transition resulting in an irreversible complex (PA'). This model can be represented by: $P + A \rightleftarrows PA \rightarrow PA'$. The second-order rate constant of the inhibition of plasmin by α_2-antiplasmin is very high (2-4×10^7 M^{-1} s^{-1}), but this high inhibition rate is dependent both upon the presence of a free lysine binding site and active site in the plasmin molecule and upon availability of a plasminogen-binding site and reactive site peptide bond in the inhibitor [16, 17]. The half-life of plasmin molecules on the fibrin surface, which have both their lysine binding sites and active site occupied, is estimated to be 2–3 orders of magnitude longer than that of free plasmin [17].

Inhibition of Plasminogen Activators by PAI-1

PAI-1 reacts very rapidly with single-chain and two-chain t-PA and with two-chain u-PA, with second-order inhibition rate constants of the order of 10^7 M^{-1} s^{-1}, but it does not react with scu-PA [18, 19].

Like other serpins, PAI-1 inhibits its target proteinases by formation of a 1:1 stoichiometric reversible complex, followed by covalent binding between the hydroxylgroup of the active site serine residue of the proteinase and the carboxylgroup of the P1 residue at the reactive center ("bait region") of the serpin. The rapid inhibition of both t-PA and u-PA by PAI-1 involves a reversible high affinity second-site interaction which does not depend on a functional active site [20]. Modeling approaches suggest that sequence 350–355 of PAI-1, which contains three negatively charged amino acids, interacts with highly positively charged regions in t-PA (residues 296–304) [21] or in u-PA (residues 179–184) [22]. In the presence of fibrin, single-chain t-PA is protected from rapid inhibition by PAI-1 [20]. It has, however, also been reported that PAI-1 binds to fibrin and that fibrin-bound PAI-1 may inhibit t-PA mediated clot lysis [23, 24].

PAI-1 occurs as an active inhibitory form that spontaneously converts to a latent form that can be partially reactivated by denaturing agents [25]. Another molecular form of intact PAI-1 has been isolated that does not form stable complexes with t-PA but is cleaved at the P1-P1' peptide bond ("substrate PAI-1") [26]. Thus, inhibitory PAI-1 may not only convert to latent PAI-1, which can be reactivated, but also to substrate PAI-1, which is irreversibly degraded by its target proteinases. This observation may thus have implications for the regulation of the fibrinolytic system.

Mechanisms Involved in Activation of the Fibrinolytic System

Plasminogen Activation by t-PA at the Fibrin Surface

t-PA is a poor enzyme in the absence of fibrin, but the presence of fibrin strikingly enhances the activation rate of plasminogen [27]. Plasmin formed at the fibrin surface has both its lysine binding sites and active site occupied and is thus only slowly inactivated by α_2-antiplasmin (half-life of about 10–100 s); in contrast, free plasmin, when formed, is rapidly inhibited by α_2-antiplasmin (half-life of about 0.1 s) [17].

During fibrinolysis, fibrinogen and fibrin itself are continuously modified by cleavage with thrombin or plasmin, yielding a diversity of reaction products [28]. Thrombin-catalyzed formation of desA-fibrin monomer, and a certain degree of desA-fibrin polymerization are essential for stimulation of plasminogen activation by t-PA. Optimal stimuation is only obtained after early plasmin-cleavage in the COOH-terminal α-chain and the NH_2-terminal β-chain of fibrin, yielding fragment X-polymer [28]. Kinetic data [27] support a mechanism in which fibrin provides a surface to which t-PA and plasminogen adsorb in a sequential and ordered way yielding a cyclic ternary complex. Formation of this complex results in an enhanced affinity of t-PA for plasminogen, yielding up to three orders of magnitude higher efficiencies for plasminogen activation. In agreement with this mechanism, the increase in fibrin stimulation after formation of fibrin X-polymers is associated with an enhanced binding of t-PA and plasminogen. This increased and altered binding of both enzyme and substrate to fibrin is mediated in part by COOH-terminal lysine residues generated by plasmin-cleavage. Interaction of these COOH-terminal lysines with lysine binding sites on t-PA and plasminogen, may allow an improved alignment as well as allosteric changes of the t-PA and plasminogen moieties, thus enhancing the rate of plasminogen activation [28].

Proteins that compete with plasminogen for binding to fibrin may have an antifibrinolytic action. Thus, Lp (a), a protein with multiple copies of a plasminogen kringle 4-like domain, a single copy of a kringle 5-like domain and an inactive proteinase domain [29], binds to fibrin via its lysine binding domains. As for plasminogen, binding of Lp (a) to fibrin is enhanced by partial proteolytic degradation of the fibrin surface [30]. Thereby, the fibrin-dependent enhancement of plasminogen activation by t-PA is reduced [31–33], although kinetic studies indicate that the effect of Lp (a) on plasminogen activation by t-PA is only very limited [34].

Alternatively, proteins that remove lysine residues from the fibrin surface, such as the Thrombin Activatable Fibrinolysis Inhibitor (TAFI) may have an antifibrinolytic action. TAFI is a 60 kDa single-chain protein, identical to plasma procarboxypeptidase B, occurring at a concentration of 75 nM [35, 36]. Thrombin, trypsin or plasmin convert the protein to an active carboxypeptidase B. Activated TAFI suppresses fibrinolysis, most likely by removing COOH-terminal lysine residues from (partially degraded) fibrin, thereby preventing additional binding of plasminogen and/or t-PA [37].

Plasminogen Activation by Staphylokinase

The *staphylokinase* gene has been cloned from the serotype B bacteriophage *sakøC*, from the serotype F bacteriophage *sak*42D and from the genomic DNA (*sak*STAR) of a staphylokinase secreting *Staphylococcus aureus* strain. It encodes a protein of 163 amino acids which is processed to a mature protein of 136 amino acids, consisting of a single polypeptide chain without disulfide bridges (for references see [38–40]).

Like streptokinase, staphylokinase is not an enzyme but it forms a 1:1 stoichiometric complex with plasmin(ogen) that activates other plasminogen molecules. When staphylokinase is added to human plasma containing of fibrin clot, it will react poorly with plasminogen in plasma, but will react with high affinity with traces of plasmin at the clot surface, converting into plasmin.staphylokinase complex which, at the clot surface, efficiently activates plasminogen to plasmin. Plasmin.staphylokinase and plasmin bound to fibrin are protected from inhibition by α_2-antiplasmin, whereas once liberated from the clot or generated in plasma, they are rapidly inhibited. Thereby the process of plasminogen activation is confined to the thrombus, preventing excessive plasmin generation, α_2-antiplasmin depletion and fibrinogen degradation in plasma (for references see [38–40]).

Plasminogen Activation by u-PA

u-PA is a serine proteinase with a high substrate-specificity for plasminogen. In contrast to tcu-PA, scu-PA displays very low activity toward low molecular weight chromogenic substrates. Scu-PA appears to have some intrinsic plasminogen activating potential, which represents 0.5% of the catalytic efficiency of tcu-PA [41, 42]. Other investigators, however, have claimed that scu-PA has no measurable intrinsic amidolytic or plasminogen activator activities [43]. The occurrence of a transitional state of scu-PA with a higher catalytic efficiency for native plasminogen than tcu-PA has been postulated [44]. Furthermore, it was reported that fibrin fragment E-2 selectively promotes the activation of plasminogen by scu-PA, mainly by enhancing the catalytic rate constant of the activation [45]. Scu-PA indeed is not an efficient activator of plasminogen bound to internal lysine residues on intact fibrin, but it develops a higher activity toward plasminogen bound to newly generated COOH-terminal lysine residues on partially degraded fibrin [46]. Subsequent studies confirmed that the fibrin-specificity of scu-PA does not require its conversion to tcu-PA, but appears to be mediated by enhanced binding of plasminogen to partially digested fibrin [47].

In plasma, in the absence of fibrin, scu-PA is stable and does not activate plasminogen; in the presence of a fibrin clot, scu-PA, but not tcu-PA, induces fibrin-specific clot lysis [41]. scu-PA does not bind to a significant extent to fibrin, although in the presence of Zn^{2+} ions some binding has been reported [48]. The intrinsic activity of scu-PA towards fibrin-bound plasminogen may contribute to its fibrin-specificity. Furthermore, α_2-antiplasmin in plasma prevents conversion of scu-PA to tcu-PA outside the clot and thus preserves fibrin-specificity [49].

Summary

One approach to the treatment of thrombosis consists of infusing thrombolytic agents to dissolve the blood clot and to restore tissue perfusion and oxygenation. Thrombolytic agents are plasminogen activators which activate the blood fibrinolytic system by activation of the proenzyme, plasminogen, to the active enzyme plasmin. Plasmin in turn digests fibrin to soluble degradation products. Inhibition of the fibrinolytic system occurs both at the level of the plasminogen activators, by plasminogen activator inhibitors (PAI-1 and PAI-2), and at the level of plasmin, mainly by α_2-antiplasmin. Streptokinase, anisoylated plasminogen streptokinase activator complex (APSAC) and two-chain urokinase-type plasminogen activator (tcu-PA) induce extensive systemic plasmin generation; α_2-antiplasmin inhibits circulating plasmin but may become exhausted during thrombolytic therapy, since its plasma concentration is only about half that of plasminogen. As a result plasmin, which has a broad substrate specificity, will degrade several plasma proteins, such as fibrinogen, coagulation factors V, VIII and XII, and von Willebrand factor. These thrombolytic agents are, therefore, considered to be non-fibrin-specific. In contrast, the physiologic plasminogen activators, tissue-type plasminogen activator (t-PA) and single-chain u-PA (scu-PA), as well as the bacterial plasminogen activator staphylokinase, are more fibrin-specific because they activate plasminogen preferentially at the fibrin surface and less in the circulation, albeit via different mechanisms. Plasmin, associated with the fibrin surface, is protected from rapid inhibition by α_2-antiplasmin because its lysine-binding sites are not available, and may thus efficiently degrade the fibrin of a thrombus.

References

1. Collen D, Lijnen HR (1991) Basic and clinical aspects of fibrinolysis and thrombolysis. Blood 78:3114–3124
2. Collen D (1997) Thrombolytic therapy. Thromb Haemost 78:742–746
3. Collen D (1996) Fibrin-selective thrombolytic therapy for acute myocardial infarction. Circulation 93:857–865

4. Forsgren M, Raden B, Israelsson M, Larsson K, Heden LO (1987) Molecular cloning and characterization of a full-length cDNA clone for human plasminogen. FEBS Lett 213:254–260

5. Collen D (1980) On the regulation and control of fibrinolysis. Thromb Haemost 43:77–89

6. Pennica D, Holmes WE, Kohr WJ, et al. (1983) Cloning and expression of human tissue-type plasminogen activator cDNA in E. coli. Nature 301:214–221

7. Lijnen HR, Collen D (1991) Strategies for the improvement of thrombolytic agents. Thromb Haemost 66:88–110

8. Holmes WE, Pennica D, Blaber M, et al. (1985) Cloning and expression of the gene for pro-urokinase in Escherichia coli. Biotechnology 3:923–929

9. Holmes WE, Nelles L, Lijnen HR, Collen D (1987) Primary structure of human alpha 2-antiplasmin, a serine protease inhibitor (serpin). J Biol Chem 262:1659–1664

10. Bangert K, Johnsen AH, Christensen U, Thorsen S (1993) Different N-terminal forms of α_2-plasmin inhibitor in human plasma. Biochem J 291:623–625

11. Wiman B, Nilsson T, Cedergren B (1982) Studies on a form of alpha 2-antiplasmin in plasma which does not interact with the lysine-binding sites in plasminogen. Thromb Res 28:193–199

12. Ichinose A, Tamaki T, Aoki N (1983) Factor XIII-mediated cross-linking of NH_2-terminal peptide of alpha2-plasmin inhibitor to fibrin. FEBS Lett 153:369–371

13. Pannekoek H, Veerman H, Lambers H, et al. (1986) Endothelial plasminogen activator inhibitor (PAI): a new member of the Serpin gene family. EMBO J 5:2539–2544

14. Declerck PJ, De Mol M, Alessi MC, et al. (1988) Purification and characterization of a plasminogen activator inhibitor-1-binding protein from human plasma. Identification as a multimeric form of S protein (vitronectin). J Biol Chem 263:15454–15461

15. Gechtman Z, Sharma R, Kreizman T, Fridkin M, Shaltiel S (1993) Synthetic peptides derived from the sequence around the plasmin cleavage site in vitronectin. Use in mapping the PAI-1 binding site. FEBS Lett 315:293–297

16. Wiman B, Collen D (1979) On the mechanism of the reaction between human α_2-antiplasmin and plasmin. J Biol Chem 254:9291–9297

17. Wiman B, Collen D (1978) On the kinetics of the reaction between human antiplasmin and plasmin. Eur J Biochem 84:573–578

18. Kruithof EKO (1988) Plasminogen activator inhibitors – a review. Enzyme 40:113–121

19. Thorsen S, Philips M, Selmer J, Lecander I, Astedt B (1988) Kinetics of inhibition of tissue-type and urokinase-type plasminogen activator by plasminogen-activator inhibitor type 1 and type 2. Eur J Biochem 175:33–39

20. Chmielewska J, Ranby M, Wiman B (1988) Kinetics of the inhibition of plasminogen activators by the plasminogen-activator inhibitor. Evidence for 'second site' interactions. Biochem J 251:327–332

21. Madison EL, Goldsmith EJ, Gerard RD, Gething MJ, Sambrook JF (1989) Serpin-resistant mutants of human tissue-type plasminogen activator. Nature 339:721–724

22. Adams DS, Griffin LA, Nachajko WR, Reddy VB, Wei CM (1991) A synthetic DNA encoding a modified human urokinase resistant to inhibition by serum plasminogen activator inhibitor. J Biol Chem 266:8476–8482

23. Wagner OF, de Vries C, Hohmann C, Veerman H, Pannekoek H (1989) Interaction between plasminogen activator inhibitor type 1 (PAI-1) bound to fibrin and either tissue-type plasminogen activator (t-PA) or urokinase-type plasminogen activator (u-PA). Binding of t-PA/PAI-1 complexes to fibrin mediated by both the finger and the kringle-2 domain of t-PA. J Clin Invest 84:647–655

24. Reilly CF, Hutzelmann JE (1992) Plasminogen activator inhibitor-1 binds to fibrin and inhibits tissue-type plasminogen activator-mediated fibrin dissolution. J Biol Chem 267:17128–17135

25. Hekman CM, Loskutoff DJ (1985) Endothelial cells produce a latent inhibitor of plasminogen activators that can be activated by denaturants. J Biol Chem 260:11581–11587

26. Declerck PJ, De Mol M, Vaughan DE, Collen D (1992) Identification of a conformationally distinct form of plasminogen activator inhibitor-1, acting as a non-inhibitory substrate for tissue-type plasminogen activator. J Biol Chem 267:11693–11696

27. Hoylaerts M, Rijken DC, Lijnen HR, Collen D (1982) Kinetics of the activation of plasmino-gen by human tissue plasminogen activator. Role of fibrin. J Biol Chem 257:2912–2919
28. Thorsen S (1992) The mechanism of plasminogen activation and the variability of the fibrin effector during tissue-type plasminogen activator-mediated fibrinolysis. Ann NY Acad Sci 667:52–63
29. McLean JW, Tomlinson JE, Kuang WJ, et al. (1987) cDNA sequence of human apolipoprotein (a) is homologous to plasminogen. Nature 330:132–137
30. Harpel PC, Gordon BR, Parker TS (1989) Plasmin catalyzes binding of lipoprotein (a) to immobilized fibrinogen and fibrin. Proc Natl Acad Sci USA 86:3847–3851
31. Fleury V, Anglès-Cano (1991) Characterization of the binding of plasminogen to fibrin sur-faces: the role of carboxy-terminal lysines. Biochemistry 30:7630–7638
32. Loscalzo J, Weinfeld M, Fless GM, Scanu AM (1990). Lipoprotein (a), fibrin binding and plas-minogen activation. Arteriosclerosis 10:240–245
33 Edelberg JM, Gonzales-Gronow M, Pizzo SV (1990) Lipoprotein (a) inhibition of plasmino-gen activation by tissue-type plasminogen activator. Thromb Res 57:155–162
34. Liu JN, Harpel PC, Pannell R, Gurewich V (1993) Lipoprotein (a): A kinetic study of its influ-ence on fibrin-dependent plasminogen activation by prourokinase or tissue plasminogen activator. Biochemistry 32:9694–9700
35. Bajzar L, Manuel R, Nesheim ME (1995) Purification and characterization of TAFI, a throm-bin-activatable fibrinolysis inhibitor. J Biol Chem 270:14477–14484
36. Eaton DL, Malloy BE, Tsai SP, Henzel W, Drayna D (1991) Isolation, molecular cloning, and partial characterization of a novel carboxypeptidase B from human plasma. J Biol Chem 266:21833–21838
37. Nesheim M, Wang W, Boffa M, Nagashima M, Morser J, Bajzar L (1997) Thrombin, thrombo-modulin and TAFI in the molecular link between coagulation and fibrinolysis. Thromb Haemost 78:386–391
38. Collen D, Lijnen HR (1994) Staphylokinase, a fibrin-specific plasminogen activator with therapeutic potential? Blood 84:680–686
39. Lijnen HR, Collen D (1996) Staphylokinase, a fibrin-specific bacterial plasminogen activator. Fibrinolysis 10:119–126
40. Collen D (1998) Staphylokinase: a potent, uniquely fibrin-selective thrombolytic agent. Nature Med 4:279–284
41. Gurewich V, Pannell R, Louie S, Kelley P, Suddith RL, Greenlee R (1984) Effective and fibrin-specific clot lysis by a zymogen precursor form of urokinase (pro-urokinase). A study in vit-ro and in two animal species. J Clin Invest 73:1731–1739
42. Lijnen HR, Van Hoef B, Nelles L, Collen D (1990) Plasminogen activation with single-chain urokinase-type plasminogen activator (scu-PA). Studies with active site mutagenized plas-minogen (Ser^{740}→Ala) and plasmin resistant scu-PA (Lys^{158}→Glu). J Biol Chem 265:5232–5236
43. Husain SS (1991) Single-chain urokinase-type plasminogen activator does not possess measurable intrinsic amidolytic or plasminogen activator activities. Biochemistry 30: 5797–5805
44. Liu J, Pannell R, Gurewich V (1992) A transitional state of pro-urokinase that has a higher catalytic efficiency against Glu-plasminogen than urokinase. J Biol Chem 267:15289–15292
45. Liu J, Gurewich V (1992) Fragment E-2 from fibrin substantially enhances pro-urokinase-induced Glu-plasminogen activation. A kinetic study using the plasmin-resistant mutant pro-urokinase Ala-158-rpro-UK. Biochemistry 31:6311–6317
46. Fleury V, Gurewich V, Anglés-Cano E (1993) A study of the activation of fibrin-bound plas-minogen by tissue-type plasminogen activator, single chain urokinase and sequential com-binations of the activators. Fibrinolysis 7:87–96
47. Fleury V, Lijnen HR, Anglés-Cano E (1993) Mechanism of the enhanced intrinsic activity of single-chain urokinase-type plasminogen activator during ongoing fibrinolysis. J Biol Chem 268:18554–18559

48. Husain SS (1993) Fibrin affinity of urokinase-type plasminogen activator. Evidence that Zn^{2+} mediates strong and specific interaction of single-chain urokinase with fibrin. J Biol Chem 268:8574–8579
49. Declerck PJ, Lijnen HR, Verstreken M, Collen D (1991) Role of α_2-antiplasmin in fibrin-specific clot lysis with single-chain urokinase-type plasminogen activator in human plasma. Thromb Haemost 65:394–398

Section III:
Functional Assessment
of the Coronary Circulation

Quantitative Echocardiographic Evaluation of Cardiac Function

J. Gorcsan III

Introduction

Echocardiographic imaging has made major contributions to the noninvasive diagnosis of cardiac structure and function. Transesophageal echocardiography (TEE) has extended the clinical utility of cardiac ultrasound to the operating room and the bedside of the critically ill patient by providing high quality two-dimensional images and Doppler data. Continued improvements in computer technology have also enabled the introduction of novel techniques to improve the quantitative analysis of cardiac function. This discussion will review traditional Doppler assessment of cardiac function by TEE, and the new technologies of automated border detection (ABD) and tissue Doppler (TD) echocardiography to assess regional and global ventricular function.

Transesophageal Doppler Assessment of Cardiac Output

Maintenance of blood flow to meet the metabolic needs of the patient is essential to survival. Cardiac output is a standard clinical measure of blood flow used as an index of left ventricular (LV) function in the intensive care unit and in the operating room. The most popular approach to calculate cardiac output is the thermodilution method that requires placement of a pulmonary artery catheter. The thermodilution method during routine usage may be highly accurate, but may be associated with complications such as vascular damage, hematoma, and pneumothorax, and even pulmonary artery rupture on rare occasion. Also, thermodilution estimates of cardiac output may be inaccurate in the presence of significant tricuspid regurgitation, and in patients with low cardiac output state.

Doppler echocardiography can estimate cardiac output and may be useful in situations where placement of a pulmonary artery catheter is not justified or where thermodilution measures are suspected to be inaccurate. The Doppler approach uses calculations of stroke volume and the following equation: Cardiac output=Stroke Volume x Heart Rate. Stroke volume measures by Doppler using both pulsed-wave and continuous-wave Doppler formats have been validated previously by transthoracic echocardiography in several studies and the same principals apply to the TEE approach [1–4]. The Doppler technique fundamentally converts shifts in received ultrasound frequency to measures of blood velocity.

Two separate types of measurements are performed to convert blood velocity data to stroke volume. The first is to estimate the cross-sectional area through which blood is flowing. This is most commonly done in the aortic annulus where geometry is circular and a measurement of diameter may be converted to circular cross-sectional area: area=1/4 π (diameter)^2.

The second measure is to integrate the blood velocity at the same site with either pulsed or continuous wave Doppler over the systolic ejection period. The integral of the spectral Doppler velocity over time, known as the flow velocity integral, is multiplied by cross-sectional area to determine stroke volume. Stroke volume is then multiplied by heart rate to determine cardiac output. Katz et al. were first to use TEE from the transgastric window to estimated cardiac output in a series of patients before and after cardiac surgery [2]. We compared Doppler measures with simultaneous thermodilution cardiac output (Fig. 1). This method utilized aortic annular diameter and assumed circular geometry for cross-sectional area and continuous-wave Doppler across the aortic valve. Aortic annular measurement can be accomplished from the mid-esophageal level in the vertical plane using a biplane probe, or 90°–120° using a multiplane probe. Doppler data are acquired from the transgastric window at 0° with a multiplane probe begin-

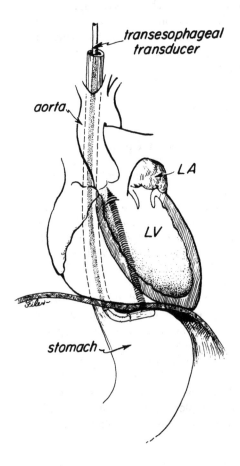

Fig. 1. Diagram of transesophageal transducer positioned to interrogate Doppler flow across the aortic valve from the transgastric window. *LA* Left atrium; *LV* left ventricle. (Reprinted with permission from [2])

ning with the mid-LV short axis view followed by extreme anteflexion and slight withdrawal to interrogate the aortic valve (Fig. 2a, b).

Continuous-wave Doppler data were available from 50 of 57 attempted studies (88%) and a close correlation of Doppler estimates with thermodilution measures was demonstrated (Fig. 3). Darmon et al. has modified this continuous-wave Doppler method from the transgastric window by using a triangular shape of the aortic orifice when calculating TEE Doppler cardiac output [4]. Data were available in 62 of 63 patients in whom many had studies before and after cardiac surgery for a total of 109 studies with a close correlation; $r=0.94$, SEE=0.4 l/min, $y=0.94x + 0.19$. These studies combine to demonstrate the accuracy of TEE Doppler estimates of cardiac output. The aortic site should probably not be used

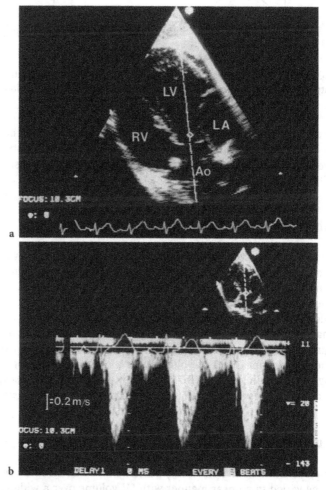

Fig. 2. a Echocardiographic image from the transgastric window with superior probe angulation to align Doppler cursor across aortic valve. *Ao* Aorta; *LA* left atrium; *LV* left ventricle; *RV* right ventricle. **b** Corresponding spectral Doppler display. (Reprinted with permission from [2])

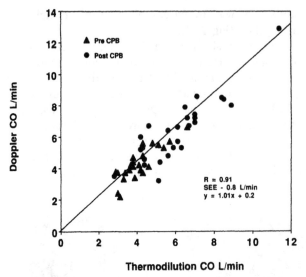

Fig. 3. Scatterplot of transesophagel Doppler estimates with thermodilution measures of cardiac output (*CO*) demonstrating close correlation. (Reprinted with permission from [2])

to estimate cardiac output in the presence of aortic stenosis, aortic regurgitation, or hypertrophic cardiomyopathy with LV outflow tract obstruction. Alternative use of the pulmonary artery or mitral valve sites may be possibly used in patients with these disorders.

Echocardiographic Automated Border Detection

The LV pressure-volume relationship has been used for many years to assess ventricular performance in a predominantly load-independent manner, however clinical applications have been limited because of technical difficulties with on-line volume acquisition [5–7]. Echocardiographic ABD has permitted the on-line calculation of two-dimensional cross-sectional cavity using backscatter signal analysis [8, 9] (Fig. 4). Multiple validation studies in animal models and in humans have demonstrated that measures of mid-LV short axis cavity area vary linearly with measures of volume over a range of physiological values. Accordingly, echocardiographic ABD has permitted the ability to assess pressure-volume relations in a less invasive manner when combined with pressure data.

Cross-Sectional Area as a Substitute for Volume

Appleyard and Glantz previously demonstrated that the mid-ventricular short-axis plane varied in a linear manner with LV volume over a wide range of alterations [10] Our group used an isolated canine heart with LV volume directly measured by a thin latex intraventricular balloon to assess the area-volume relationship using

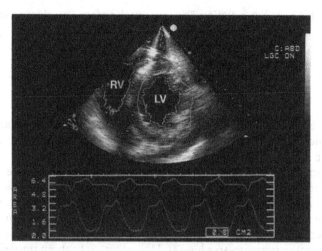

Fig. 4. Echocardiographic image from the mid-ventricular short axis plane demonstrating automated border detection measurement of cross-sectional cavity area in real time from a patient undergoing transesophageal echocardiography. *LV* Left ventricle; *RV* right ventricle. (Reprinted with permission72:721 from [13])

ABD [11]. Reproducibly linear relationships were shown over the physiological range of values. A study in an open chest dog with an intact circulation revealed linear correlations with changes in cross-sectional area by ABD and stroke volume by an electromagnetic flow probe placed on the ascending aorta as a standard of reference [12]. Subsequent studies in humans demonstrated similar linear relationships between ABD measures of LV cross-sectional area and electromagnetic flow probe measures of LV ejection volume, and radionuclide ejection fraction [13–15]. These studies and others combined to support the use of LV cross-sectional area as a surrogate for LV volume when assessing pressure-volume relations.

Left Ventricular Pressure-Area Relations

Assessment of LV performance using ABD pressure-area relations was made possible by a customized interface with the ABD echocardiography system (Hewlett-Packard, Andover, MA). This interface permitted the output of the LV cavity area signal to be interfaced with an analog-to-digital converter and recorded on a computer [15–16]. A plot of area and pressure could be programmed to display pressure-area loops in real time. Timing adjustment of pressure-area loops was occasionally necessary because of the fixed frame rate of the ABD ultrasound system at 30 Hz. The timing of the area waveform was shifted to align the point before the onset of isovolumic contraction on the pressure signal with the first occurrence of maximal ABD area [15, 16]. Previously described calculations from pressure-volume loops were then applied to the pressure-area loops as a means to assess contractility [5–7]. These equations were applied to a series of pressure-area loops over a wide range in values that were induced by inferior vena caval occlusions in our studies. The end-systolic pressure-volume relationship (ESPVR) or end-systolic elastance (Ees) was calculated as the slope of the maximal pressure/area point for each beat using an iterative linear regression technique. Time-varying elastance was also solved using the equation:

$$E(t) = P(t)/[A(t) - Ao(t)]$$

where E=elastance, P=pressure, t=time, A=Area, Ao=Area axis intercept. Elastance or the slope of the pressure-area relations was then plotted over time with the maximal value as Emax. Preload recruitable stroke work was also calculated from the pressure-area loops as an alternative load insensitive means to assess LV performance [17]. Stroke work values from individual beats were then plotted vs. the corresponding end-diastolic area values and linear regression analysis define the slope of this relationship as preload recruitable stroke work [14]. The preload recruitable stroke work approach has the advantage of using information from the entire pressure-area loop and the uncertainty about the definition of end-systole was avoided. Estimates of Ees, Emax and preload recruitable stroke work were used to demonstrate alterations in contractility induced by inotropic modulation. Predicted increases were induced by low dose dobutamine infusion (2–5 µg/kg/min) and decreases were induced by the induction of heart failure by high doses of the β-blocker propranolol (2–5 mg bolus) (Fig. 5). Arterial pressure may be used as a substitute for LV pressure to plot pressure-area loops [18, 19]. This method can yield similar estimates of Ees when adjusted for the delay in timing associated with arterial pressure (Fig. 6). The use of arterial pressure may likely expand the clinical use of ABD pressure area-relations.

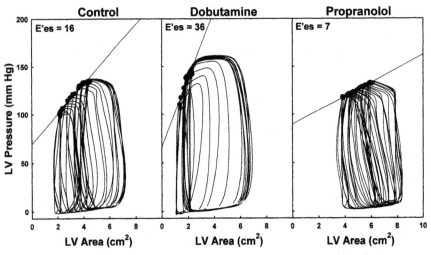

Fig. 5. Examples of pressure-area loops over a range of values induced by inferior vena caval occlusions from a canine model. Representative loops from control conditions and inotropic modulation with dobutamine and propranolol are shown. Alterations in end-systolic elastance (*E'es*) are demonstrated indicating respective changes in contractility. (Reprinted with permission of the American College of Cardiology from [22])

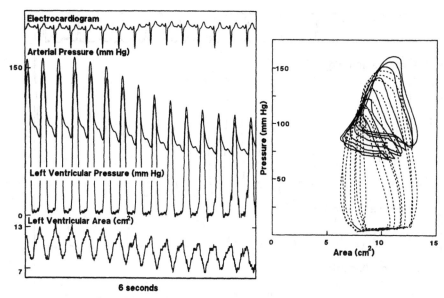

Fig. 6. Examples of waveform data (*left*) and pressure-area loop data (*right*) during an inferior vena caval occlusion in a patient before bypass surgery. *Solid line* arterial pressure-area loops; *dashed line* simultaneous left ventricular pressure-area loops. (Reprinted with permission from [18])

Preload Adjusted Maximal Power

Power is defined as the rate at which work is done and is usually expressed in units of Watts. Power can be expressed as the product of pressure and flow in a hemodynamic system. Kass and co-workers have recently demonstrated that power can be used as a load insensitive means to assess LV function by mathematically adjusting for effects of preload by dividing by (end-diastolic volume)^2, known as preload adjusted maximal power (PA-PWR$_{max}$) [20, 21]. We have recently expanded this concept to assess LV contractility using ABD echocardiography [22]. Power was calculated by multiplying simultaneous LV pressure by the first derivative of the ABD LV area signal (dA/dt) as an estimate of flow. We demonstrated that power calculations were insensitive to changes in afterload (Fig. 7). However, preload adjustment was required because of the affects of preload on power. The best correction factor of several tested was ÷ (end-diastolic area)$^{3/2}$. Accordingly, relatively load insensitive estimates of LV function using ABD cross-sectional area as a surrogate for LV volume could be expressed as:

$$PA\text{-}PWR_{max} = PWR_{max}/(\text{end-diastolic area})^{3/2}$$

PA-PWR$_{max}$ was able to demonstrated predictable changes in contractility induced by pharmacological inotropic modulation (Fig. 8). Furthermore, arterial pressure could be substituted for LV ejection pressure, which adds promise as a less invasive method. The major advantage of power calculations over pressure-

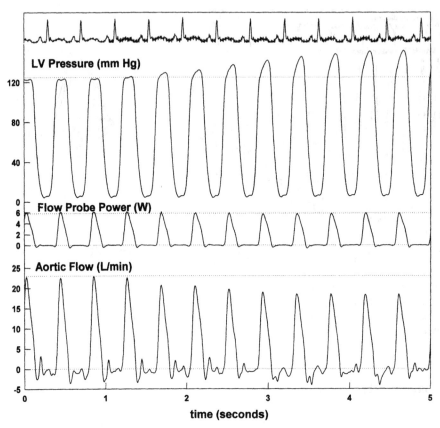

Fig. 7. Waveform plots of left ventricular (*LV*) pressure, aortic flow from an electromagnetic flow probe, and corresponding power calculation during increases in afterload induced aortic occlusion in a canine model. The afterload insensivity of power is shown. (Reprinted with permission of the American College of Cardiology from [22])

volume or pressure-area loop calculations is that this measure can be made during baseline conditions and acute alteration of loading is not required. Further testing of PA-PWR$_{max}$ using ABD in humans studies is in progress [23].

Tissue Doppler Echocardiography

Tissue Doppler (TD) is recent modification of the color Doppler technique that fundamentally utilizes ultrasound frequency shifts to calculate velocity. TD, unlike routine color flow Doppler, focuses on the comparatively lower velocity range of tissue motion and is extends the diagnostic capabilities of echocardiography to quantify LV function. Routine color flow instrumentation also uses the autocorrelator technique to calculate and display color-coded blood velocity along a series of ultrasound scan lines within a two-dimensional sector. Color

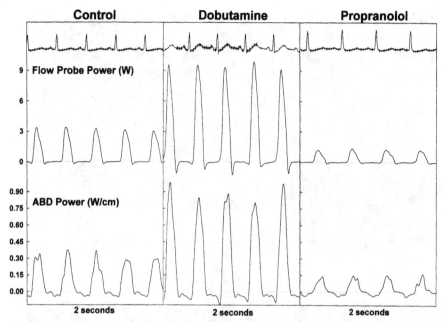

Fig. 8. Alterations in power induced by positive inotropic modulation with dobutamine and negative inotropic modulation with propranolol. Similar results are seen with flow probe power and echocardiographic automated border detection (*ABD*). Reprinted with permission of the American College of Cardiology from [22])

flow Doppler-imaging instrumentation commonly employs a high pass filter to block out the low velocity Doppler shifts created by tissue motion and enhances the display of blood velocity. TD is a modification of this technique by bypassing this high pass filter and inputting low velocity Doppler shift data directly into the autocorrelator [24–26]. Color-coded tissue velocities are then superimposed on conventional M-mode and two-dimensional images (Fig. 9). An advantage of TD is that Doppler shifts of tissue motion are of high amplitude with favorable signal-to-noise ratios [26–28].

Validation of Tissue Doppler Measures

Validation studies have demonstrated that TD can accurately reflect tissue velocity. Yamazaki et al. reported an in vitro experimental model where TD imaged an acoustic reflection board that was moving uniformly with a known velocity in a water bath [25]. TD color M-mode measured velocity accurately from –40–40 mm/s; r=0.99, SEE=8 mm/s, y=0.99x + 0.54. A second in vitro study was reported by Miyatake et al. where a foam disc was rotated with a known rotational velocity in a water bath while being imaged by two-dimensional TD [26]. TD was able to accurately measure velocity in B-mode of display while correcting for the Doppler angle of incidence; r=0.99, y=0.97 x + 2.17 for linear regression of 23

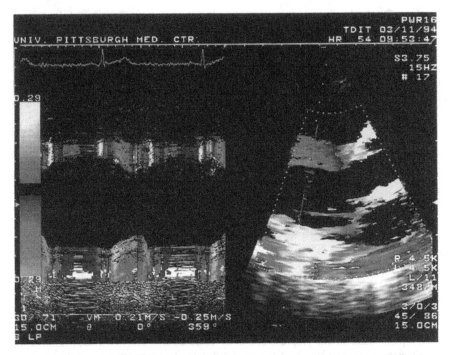

Fig. 9. Tissue Doppler echocardiographic image from a normal subject demonstrating color-coded two-dimensional image on right and corresponding color M-mode on left. Myocardial velocity is color-coded. (Reprinted with permission from [27])

measures from – 10–10 cm/s. The ability of TD to measure endocardial velocity in humans has also been reported by comparing TD velocity values to estimates of velocity from digitized routine M-modes scans. Peak velocity measured by TD correlated closely with peak velocity by digitized M-modes in a series of 27 subjects; $r=0.99$, $y=0.94x + 0.64$. Posterior wall endocardial velocities throughout the cardiac cycle by TD were shown to correlate with velocity estimated from digitized M-modes in 16 subjects with a group mean results as follows: $r=0.88\pm0.03$, SEE=6.9$\pm$1.1 mm/s, $y=0.70 x + 1.9\pm1.5$ mm/s [27]. Similar favorable observations have also been reported by other groups [29–31].

Quantification of Regional Left Ventricular Function

Traditional assessment of regional LV function is accomplished by visual interpretation of endocardial excursion and wall thickening which is subjective. TD research has focused on using measures of myocardial velocity to quantify regional wall motion. We performed a study in an animal model to evaluate endocardial velocity by TD using a commercially available ultrasound system (SSA–380 A, Toshiba Corp., Tochigi, Japan) as a means to objectively quantify alterations in regional contractility over a wide range induced by inotropic modulation [32]. High fidelity pressure and conductance catheters were used to assess LV contractility in a predominantly load-independent manner by pressure-volume relations in an open-chest dog model. Mid-LV M-mode and two-dimensional color TD images were recorded during control and inotropic modulation stages with dobutamine and esmolol as positive and negative inotropes, respectively. Group mean TD peak endocardial systolic velocity increased significantly with infusion of 4 µg/kg/min dobutamine from 4.5±1.8–7.2±1.9* cm/s and decreased with infusion of 650±50 µg/kg/min esmolol from 4.4±1.6–2.8±1.5*cm/s, (*p<0.01 vs. control; Fig. 10). The group mean end-systolic pressure-volume relation increased from 2.06±0.50–4.86±1.75* mmHG/ml with dobutamine and decreased with esmolol from 2.07±0.56–1.61±0.91* mmHG/ml. Changes in TD peak systolic velocity were correlated significantly with changes in contractility measured by the end-systolic pressure-volume relations (r=0.85±0.04). These data from this animal model demonstrate that TD measures reflect directional and incremental alterations in LV contractility and have potential to quantify regional LV function.

Our group has applied TD to quantify regional LV function using TD time-velocity plots in a pilot series of 12 patients with known LV dysfunction: 10 from myocardial infarction and 2 from idiopathic dilated cardiomyopathy [26]. Anteroseptal and posterior wall endocardial time-velocity plots were constructed from TD color M-modes on these patients and compared to a series of 20 normal control subjects. TD was able to quantify abnormal segmental function with peak systolic velocity being significantly lower in abnormal anteroseptal and posterior wall segments compared to normal control (Fig. 11). Furthermore, the TD systolic endocardial velocity data correlated significantly with measures of percentage wall thickening from routine two-dimensional imaging (Fig. 12). These studies and data from other groups combine to demonstrate the clinical potential to quantify regional LV function by TD.

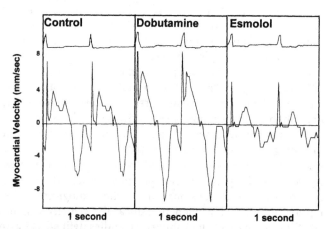

Fig. 10. Endocardial time-velocity plots from tissue Doppler data in an open-chest dog model during inotropic modulation with dobutamine and esmolol demonstrating corresponding increases and decreases in myocardial function

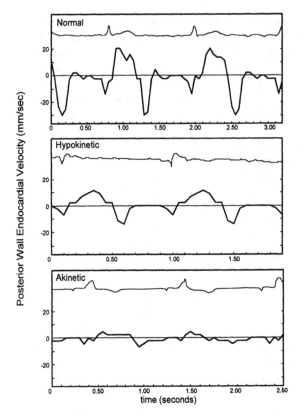

Fig. 11. Tissue Doppler posterior wall endocardial time-velocity plots in from a normal subject (*top*), a patient with coronary artery disease and posterior hypokinesis (*middle*) and a patient with a posterior wall myocardial infarction (*bottom*). (Reprinted with permission from [27])

Dobutamine Stress Echocardiography

Previous studies have observed an ischemic cascade where segmental LV dysfunction may occur with myocardial ischemia before either electrocardiographic changes or angina pectoris. This concept has served as the basis of stress echocardiographic imaging to detect early signs of ischemia [33, 34]. Although stress echocardiographic interpretation has demonstrated an average sensitivity of 89%, specificity of 80% and the overall accuracy of 87% for detecting angiographically significant coronary artery disease, visual interpretation of wall motion abnormalities remains subjective [35]. The feasibility of TD was tested to more objectively assess regional LV function during dobutamine stress echocardiography in a study of 55 patients using standard dobutamine stress protocols up to 50 µg/kg/min. Paired routine and TD images were acquired from standard views [36]. Twenty-two patients reached their target heart rate with normal routine two-dimensional stress echocardiograms and served as a control group for the normal segmental endocardial velocity response to dobutamine stress. Nineteen patients had abnormal studies defined as having hypokinetic or akinetic segments at peak stress by routine two-dimensional criteria. For 114 segments pooled from the parasternal views, endocardial velocity in abnormal

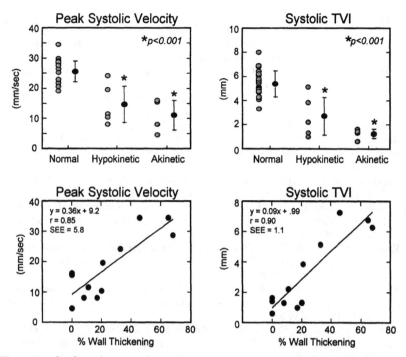

Fig. 12. Tissue Doppler data of groups of normal subjects and patients with abnormal posterior wall function showing alterations in peak systolic velocity and systolic time-velocity integral (*TVI*) than correlate with % wall thickening. Reprinted with permission from [27])

segments at peak stress was 3.0±1.4 cm/s compared to 7.2±1.8 cm/s in the normal control group (*P*<0.05 vs. control). Similar results were observed in basal and mid segments from the apical four chamber view at peak stress with peak endocardial velocity being 3.7±1.5 cm/s in 113 abnormal segments versus 7.6±1.9 cm/s in the corresponding control segments (*P*<0.05 vs. control). However, the peak endocardial velocity response in abnormal apical segments was not significantly different from control values, and represents a limitation of this method. Excluding apical segments, a maximum velocity of <5.5 cm/s at peak stress was able to identify abnormal segments with average sensitivity of 96%, specificity of 81%, and accuracy of 86%. This study demonstrates that TD has potential to increase the quantitative approach to interpretation of dobutamine stress echocardiography.

This discussion has reviewed only a few of the exciting new technological advances in echocardiography that have enhanced our ability to quantify LV function. These methods are in evolution as further refinements and enhancements continue to progress. Clinical applications of these echocardiographic techniques will likely continue to expand to future settings.

References

1. Gorcsan J, Diana P, Ball BA, Hattler BG. (1992) Intraoperative determination of cardiac output by transesophageal continuous wave Doppler. Am Heart J 123:171–176
2. Katz WE, Gasior TA, Quinlan JJ, Gorcsan J. (1993) Transgastric continuous-wave Doppler to determine cardiac output. Am J Cardiol 71:853–857
3. Stoddard MF, Prince CR, Ammish N, Goad JL, Vogel RL. (1993) Pulsed Doppler transesophageal echocardiographic determination of cardiac output in human beings: Comparison with thermodilution technique. Am Heart J 126:956–962
4. Darmon PL, Hillel Z, Mogtader A, Mindich B, Thys D. (1994) Cardiac Output by transesophageal echocardiography using continuous-wave Doppler across the aortic valve. Anesthesiology 80:796–805
5. Suga H, Sagawa K. (1974) Instantaneous pressure-volume relationships and their ratio in the excised, supported canine left ventricle. Circ Res 35:117–126
6. Little WC, Freeman GL, O'Rourke RA. (1985) Simultaneous determination of left ventricular end-systolic pressure-volume and pressure-dimension relationships in closed-chest dogs. Circulation 6:1301–1308
7. Kass DA, Yamazaki T, Burkhoff D, Maughan WL, Sagawa K. (1986) Determination of left ventricular end-systolic pressure-volume relationships by the conductance (volume) catheter technique. Circulation 3:586–595
8. Perez JE, Waggoner AD, Barzilai B, Melton HE, Miller JG, Sobel BE. (1992) On-line assessment of ventricular function by automatic boundary detection and ultrasonic backscatter imaging. J Am Coll Cardiol 19:313–320
9. Vandenberg BF, Rath LS, Stuhlmuller P, Melton HE, Skorton D. (1992) Estimation of left ventricular cavity area with an on-line semiautomated echocardiographic edge detection system. Circulation 86:159–166
10. Appleyard RF, Glantz SA. Two-dimensions describe left ventricular volume change during hemodynamic transients. Am J Physiol 1990, 258:H277-H284
11. Gorcsan J, Morita S, Mandarino WA, et al. (1993) Two-dimensional echocardiographic automated border detection accurately reflects changes in left ventricular volume. J Am Soc Echocardiogr 6:482–489
12. Gorcsan J, Lazar JM, Romand J, Pinsky MR. (1993) On-line estimation of stroke volume by means of echocardiographic automated border detection in the canine left ventricle. Am Heart J 125:1316–1323
13. Gorcsan J, Gasior TA, Mandarino WA, Deneault LG, Hattler BG, Pinsky MR. (1993) On-line estimation of changes in left ventricular stroke volume by transesophageal echocardiograhic automated border detection in patients undergoing coronary artery bypass grafting. Am J Cardiol 72:721–72
14. Gorcsan J, Lazar JM, Schulman DS, Follansbee WP. (1993) Comparison of left ventricular function by echocardiographic automated border detection and by radionuclide ejection fraction. Am J Cardiol 72:810–815
15. Gorcsan J, Romand JA, Mandarino WA, Deneault LG, Pinsky MR. (1994) Assessment of left ventricular performance by on-line pressure-area relations using echocardiographic automated border detection. J Am Coll Cardiol 23:242–252
16. Gorcsan J, Gasior TA, Mandarino WA, Deneault LG, Hattler BG, Pinsky MR. (1994) Assessment of the immediate effects of cardiopulmonary bypass on left ventricular performance by on-line pressure-area relations. Circulation 89:180–190
17. Glower DD, Spratt, JA, Snow ND, et al. (1985) Linearity of the Frank-Starling relationship in the intact heart: the concept of preload recruitable stroke work. Circulation 5:994–1009
18. Gorcsan J, Denault A, Gasior et al. (1994) Rapid estimation of left ventricular contractility from end-systolic relations by echocardiographic automated border detection and femoral arterial pressure. Anesthesiology 81:553–562

19. Denault AY, Gorcsan J, Mandarino WA, Kancel MJ, Pinsky MR. (1997) End-systolic relations using echocardiographic automated border detection and arterial pressure to assess left ventricular performance. Am J Physiol 272;H138-H147

20. Kass DA, Beyer R. (1991) Evaluation of contractile state by maximal ventricular power divided by the square of end-diastolic volume. Circulation 84:1698-1708

21. Sharir T, Feldman MD, Haber H et al. (1994) Ventricular systolic assessment in patients with dilated cardiomyopathy by preload-adjusted maximal power: Validation and noninvasive application. Circulation 89:2045-2053

22. Mandarino WA, Pinsky MR, Gorcsan J. (1998) Assessment of left ventricular contractile state by preload-adjusted maximal power using echocardiographic automated border detection. J Am Coll Cardiol 31:861-868

23. Mahler CM, Katz WE, Murali S, Feldman MD, Gorcsan J. (1996) Preload-adjusted maximal power using echocardiographic automated border detection to assess left ventricular function. J Am Coll Cardiol, 50 A (abst)

24. Sutherland GR, Stewart MJ, Groundstroem KWE, et al. (1994) Color Doppler Myocardial Imaging: A new technique for assessment of myocardial function. J Am Soc Echocardiogr 7:441-58

25. Yamazaki N, Mine Y, Sano A, et al. (1994) Analysis of ventricular wall motion using color-coded tissue Doppler imaging system. Jpn J Appl Phys 33:3141-3146

26. Miyatake K, Yamagishi M, Tanaka N, et al. (1995) New method of evaluating left ventricular wall motion by color-coded tissue Doppler imaging: In vitro and in vivo studies. J Am Coll Cardiol 25:717-724

27. Gorcsan J, Gulati, VK, Mandarino WA, Katz WE. (1996) Color-coded measures of myocardial velocity throughout the cardiac cycle by tissue Doppler imaging to quantify regional left ventricular function. Am Heart J 131:1203-1213

28. Gulati VK, Katz WE, Follansbee WP, Gorcsan J. (1996) Mitral annular descent velocity by tissue Doppler echocardiography as an index of global left ventricular function. Am J Cardiol 77:979-984

29. Fleming AD, Xia X, McDicken WN, Sutherland GR, Fenn L. (1994) Myocardial velocity gradients detected by Doppler imaging. Br J Radiol 67:679-688

30. Palka P, Lange A, Sutherland GR, Fleming AD, Fenn L, McDicken WN. (1995) Doppler tissue imaging: Myocardial wall motion velocities in normal subjects. J Am Soc Echocardiogr 8:659-668

31. Donovan LD, Armstrong WF, Bach DS. (1995) Quantitative Doppler tissue imaging of the left ventricular myocardium: Validation in normal subjects. Am Heart J 130:100-104

32. Gorcsan J, Strum D, Mandarino WA, Gulati V, Pinsky MR. (1997) Quantitative assessment of alterations in regional left ventricular contractility by tissue Doppler echocardiography: Comparison with sonomicrometry and pressure-volume relations. Circulation 95:2423-2433

33. Sawada SG, Segar DS, Ryan T, et al. (1991) Echocardiographic detection of coronary artery disease during dobutamine infusion. Circulation 83:1605-14

34. Pellikka PA, Roger VL, Oh JK, Miller FA, Seward JB, Tajik J. (1995) Stress echocardiography. Part II. Dobutamine stress echocardiography: Techniques, implementation, clinical applications, and correlations. Mayo Clin Proc 70:16-27

35. Hoffmann R, Lethen H, Marwick T, et al. (1996) Analysis of interinstitutional observer agreement in interpretation of dobutamine stress echocardiograms. J Am Coll Cardiol 27:330-6

36. Katz WE, Gulati VK, Mahler CM, Gorcsan J. (1997) Quantitative evaluation of the segmental left ventricular response to dobutamine stress by tissue Doppler echocardiography. Am J Cardiol 79:1036-1042

Prognosis in Unstable Angina

J. Figueras

Introduction

Unstable angina has always encompassed a variety of conditions that have interfered with a linear evaluation of its natural course since patients with prolonged history of stable angina have been evaluated along with those of recent onset angina and those with prolonged angina and persistent ST-T wave changes [1-12]. Surprisingly enough, the tendency has been to enlarge the group with patients with a non-Q wave myocardial infarction which in itself includes also a rather broad spectrum of conditions such as a transmural posterior myocardial necrosis or an extensive subendocardial infarction [1, 2, 4-6, 12]. The reason for such a broad concept is the knowledge of a likely common underlying physiopathology [1, 2, 4-6, 12]. In fact, cases with either a recent onset angina at rest, a progressive stable angina or a prolonged angina, with or without enzyme elevation, appear to have in common a fractured plaque [13-16] with a thrombotic component of variable size, which causes a critical coronary stenosis or a temporary occlusion [1, 2, 4-6, 12]. Presumably, the determinants of the in-hospital course of these different presentations could be the same as those that may condition their initial follow-up after discharge. Nevertheless, the term "unstable" is still presiding this syndrome because of the uncertainty of the in-hospital course which may eventually lead to an infarction or a reinfarction, a cardiac death or to the need for in-hospital coronary revascularization.

Natural History

To describe the natural history of unstable angina, term first coined by Fowler [17] although the condition had been previously defined as preinfarction angina, reference has to be addressed to clinical series preceding coronary bypass grafting [18-20] or to those of institutions inclined to conservative management [21] or to studies in which both therapeutic alternatives were randomized [22]. Clearly, long-term follow-up of medically managed patients is almost nonexistent because of the crossover of refractory patients to coronary revascularization.

Most studies on unstable angina include patients with recent onset angina at rest or elicited by little efforts, those with a progressive exercise-induced angina, associated or not to rest angina, or cases of prolonged angina, longer than 30 min, that occurs generally at rest [14, 18, 19, 22–30]. Fortunately, and in spite of the challenging title of an unstable syndrome, most patients, 60–80%, gain clinical stability with bed rest and medical therapy within the first 2–3 days [14, 18, 19, 22–30]. The incidence of myocardial infarction is about 8–10% within the first 30 days [14, 18, 19, 22–32] and, in general, infarct size is small to moderate and except for patients with postinfarction angina [30, 33–35], its prognosis is not grave. In-hospital or first month mortality is about 3–5% [18, 19, 22–32, 36] but it may range from zero to 8% depending upon the kind of patients included. In this regard, the worse series for incidence of infarction (17%) and mortality (8%) was that of Gazes et al. [18], one of the pioneering studies. Mortality is mostly related to development of infarction, coronary surgery and, in a few patients, is produced by a sudden electromechanical dissociation [30, 37]. Although the rate of these complications has been in part reduced by the use of aspirin and heparin [29, 36] recent reports have found an still high incidence [32, 38] in spite of these therapies. Some of them observing no differences between aspirin alone or combined with heparin [38] while other recent smaller series encounter a lower incidence [36, 39–41].

In the first 6 months of follow-up the incidence of infarction ranges from 3% to 13% [23, 26, 42] and at 1 year is close to 13% [19, 28]. In most of these series mortality at 3–6 months was 3–4% [23, 26, 42] and at 1 year between 10% and 18% [18, 19, 22, 23, 28, 42].

Prognostic Markers

Factors that are known to be associated with an increased incidence of events are the presence of extensive coronary artery disease [16, 22, 24, 30, 34, 43–45], the recurrence of anginal or silent ischemic episodes [7, 18, 21, 24, 25, 30, 46], the presence of electrocardiographic changes during pain [7, 18, 30, 44], and the presence of enzyme elevation [4, 30, 34, 35, 47, 48], even when mild, or of a reduced coronary reserve [30], the latter mostly referring to early follow-up prognosis [49–55].

Recurrence of Angina

The negative prognostic value of persistence of symptoms, particularly beyond the first 48 h, was already noticed by Gazes et al. with respect to the in-hospital and 1-year mortality [18]. This had also a bearing on the incidence of infarction as shown by Mulcahy who observed that in patients without recurrent symptoms incidence of infarction was 2% whereas in those with persistent symptoms during 6 days or beyond the 6th day was of 10% and of 26%, respectively [21]. Likewise, Olson et al. documented that in a series of 193 among those with recurrent angina beyond the first 24 h, the incidence of infarction at 2 years was of 15% and mortality of 32%, while in those without angina it was of 8% and 7% respectively [7]. Among others, we have recently confirmed that among 383 patients with unstable angina, those who died or experienced a myocardial infarction during hospitalization had twice as much anginal episodes than those who presented none [30].

Although in smaller series, the prognostic value of the presence of silent myocardial ischemia as detected by Holter monitoring has also shown coincidental results with those associated with recurrent angina, both in the in-hospital and in the follow-up prognosis [24, 25, 46, 56, 57]. Gottlieb et al. observed that among 70 patients those with silent ischemia had a higher incidence of infarction (16% vs. 3%) and of need for revascularization (27% vs. 10%) than those without ischemia [25]. Similarly, Nadamanee [46] and Bugiardini [58] documented that patients with prolonged periods of silent ischemia, longer than 60 min, had a greater need for early revascularization.

Electrocardiographic Changes and During Angina

In addition to recurrent angina, the presence or absence of electrocardiographic changes during pain have also relevant prognostic implications. Accordingly, Gazes's observations had already indicated a greater incidence of infarction and mortality at 3 months among patients with ST segment depression during angina than in those without changes [18], and Olson also observed that among those with angina the subset with transient electrocardiographic changes had a higher infarction (42% vs. 17%) and mortality rates (21% vs. 7%) than in those without changes [7]. Furthermore, De Servi et al. indicated that among 416 patients, all with ECG changes during pain, the incidence of infarction was higher among patients who presented ST segment elevation during angina at rest than those with ST segment depression (15% vs. 6%) but mortality was higher in the latter subset (3.2% vs. 0.5%) [44]. In our series, we appreciated that patients without ECG changes during angina presented absence of in-hospital infarction or mortality whereas those with ECG changes had a mortality and an infarction rates of 5.6% and 19%, respectively [30]. Moreover, and as in the series of Gazes [18], patients with ST segment depression had the highest incidence of these complications [30]. More recent studies have largely confirmed these results [59].

Extent of Coronary Artery Disease

The coronary angiographic findings are of considerable prognostic value [16, 22, 24, 30, 34, 43–45]. This association was initially indicated by Allison in a series of 188 patients who observed that of the 7 patients who died, 6 had severe stenosis of the left main and one had multivessel disease [16]. Russell also reported that the incidence of infarction in patients with triple vessel disease was twice as much that of single vessel disease during hospitalization, and a sixfold higher during the first year of follow-up [22]. Similarly, in our series the incidence of infarction in patients with multivessel disease was nearly twice that of single vessel disease and the in-hospital mortality was sevenfold larger [30]. In addition to the number of vessels critically stenosed, some investigators have claimed that the kind of morphology of the culprit stenosis may also have prognostic implications [34]. In this regard, Bugiardini et al. have postulated that complex lesions have a worse prognosis than uncomplicated lesions. However, in their series predominated patients with postinfarction angina [43%], a condition known to be bound to a higher rate of thrombosis and complicated lesions [34]. Other investigators, however, have found no relationship between the kind of lesion and the occurrence of in-hospital events [60].

Although a reduced ejection fraction seems to be associated with a higher incidence of complications [45], the sensitivity of this finding is low because most patients with unstable angina have an ejection fraction above 50% [30, 34, 45, 61].

Elevated Enzymes

The presence of even a modest increase in myocardial enzymes is associated with a higher infarction and mortality rates during hospitalization [4, 30, 34, 48] and in the follow-up [35, 47]. This was already pointed out using the values of MB creatine phosphokinase [4, 24, 30, 34] and more recently similar findings have been described with the use of Troponin T [48]. Perhaps too much emphasis has been lately placed in this marker for if these patients are to be considered as having had a non-wave myocardial infarction one would expect to have a similar in-hospital and follow-up course [62, 63]. Amstrong observed that by examining the MB creatine phosphokinase every 4 h in 199 patients with unstable angina, the 38 who presented a slight or moderate rise had a 1-year mortality twice than that of patients without enzyme rise [24]. We also encountered that in this subset of patients, 84 of 383 (22%), the incidence of in hospital serious events (infarction, death, or surgical coronary revascularization) was nearly twofold that of patients without enzyme rise (30% vs. 19%, $P<0.05$) [30].

Coronary Reserve: Stress Test

Several studies have documented the prognostic value of a discharge positive exercise stress test for the occurrence of ischemic events in the follow-up in patients with unstable angina [49–52]. Nixon observed that a positive submaximal stress test 3 days after the last anginal episode was associated with a higher rate of hospital readmissions for unstable angina [49]. Swahn reported that in 394 patients, a predischarge positive submaximal bicycle stress test was associated with a higher incidence of death, myocardial infarction or surgical revascularization at 1 year than those with a negative test (40% vs. 2.5%) [51]. Likewise, Butman observed that among 125 patients those with a positive stress test 4 days after stabilization had a higher incidence of severe angina (28% vs. 3%), a higher rate of readmission for unstable angina (15% vs 5%) or a higher need for surgical revascularization (37% vs. 17%) during 1 year of follow-up than those with a negative test [50]. More recently, the presence of myocardial ischemia in a scintigraphic exercise test, also prior to discharge, has also been shown to be associated with a higher rate of complications in the follow-up [54, 55, 64].

In our study we assessed coronary reserve using atrial pacing to examine the in-hospital rather than the follow-up prognostic value of this marker [30]. We observed that a reduced coronary reserve (ST segment shift 1 mm at 140–150 beats/min) was associated with a higher rates of in-hospital death (3.8% vs. 0.6%) or myocardial infarction (12.4% vs. 2.6%) than those with a normal reserve [30]. Moreover, this event rate was even higher in those with a lower pacing ischemic threshold (130 beats/min, 6.9% and 18.4%, respectively, $p<0.001$) [30]. Therefore, measurement of coronary reserve is not only of prognostic value for the follow-up of patients with unstable angina, as it is for those with stable angina [47, 65, 66], but also for in-hospital events.

General Comments

It is nowadays accepted that the condition of unstable angina is associated with an acutely complicated arteriosclerotic plaque with the formation of a local thrombus and a consequent reduction of coronary lumen to a critical level [5, 12]. In these circumstances, small increments of myocardial oxygen consumption related to mild exercise and/or further reductions in coronary blood flow at the culprit lesion by local vasoconstriction and/or by transient increases in the size of the thrombus, seem a plausible explanation for the decline in ischemic threshold and the appearance and recurrence of spontaneous pain at rest [5, 12, 24, 30]. In this physiopathological setting, subsequent development of infarction or death, mostly caused also by occlusion at the culprit lesion, would depend on the course of phenomena occurring at the complicated plaque. Theoretically, therefore, factors such as the extent of coronary artery disease and a reduced coronary reserve would have little bearing in the in-hospital outcome of these patients. Nevertheless, and for unclear reasons these two factors are, consistently, the most relevant ones in terms of prognosis [30, 42–45]. Therefore, the parallelism between unstable angina [30, 49–52] and stable angina [49, 65, 66] with respect to these main prognostic markers in spite of their different pathogenesis of the ischemic episodes, is noteworthy. This coincidental prognostic value is particularly striking with respect to mortality. In fact, cardiogenic shock associated with acute myocardial infarction, which is the most common form of death in the two settings, is largely associated with advanced coronary disease. Thus, patients with a reduced coronary reserve are particularly vulnerable to the ischemic episodes presenting a higher rate of heart failure than those with a more preserved coronary reserve. The incidence of infarction is also related to these two factors but to a lesser extent which may explain that, in at least some instances, the importance of a reduced thrombolytic capacity [67, 68] and/or an increased prothrombotic status. Recently, some investigators have underscored the possible role of inflammation in the in-hospital prognosis of these patients mainly relying on the levels of reactive protein C [68, 69].

The increased risk of complications in patients with ST segment depression during pain may be accounted for their association with a more extensive coronary disease and a more compromised coronary reserve than those with ST segment elevation.

References

1. Dalen JE, Ockene IS, Alpert JS. Coronary spasm, coronary thrombosis and myocardial infarction: a hypothesis concerning the pathophysiology of acute myocardial infarction. Am Heart J 1982; 104: 1119–1124.
2. Mandelkorn JB, Wolf NM, Singh S, Schechter JA, Kersh RI, Rodgers DM, Workman MB, Bentivoglio LG, LaPorte SM, Meister SG. Intracoronary thrombi in nontransmural infarction and unstable angina. Am J Cardiol 1983; 52: 1–6.
3. Gohlke H, Samek L, Betz P, Roskam H. Exercise testing provides additional prognostic information in angiographically defined subgroups of patients with coronary artery disease. Circulation 1983; 68: 979–985.
4. Boden WE, Bough EW, Benham I, Shulman RS. Unstable angina with episodic ST segment elevation with minimal creatine kinase release culminating in extensive recurrent infarction. J Am Coll Cardiol 1983; 2: 11–20.
5. Ambrose JA, Hjemdahl-Monsen CE, Borrico S, Gorlin R, Fuster V. Angiographic demonstration of a common link between unstable angina pectoris and non-Q-wave myocardial infarction. Am J Cardiol 1988; 61: 244–247.
6. Schreiber TL, Macina G, McNulty A, Bunnell P, Kikel M, Miller DM, Devereux RB, Tenney R, Cowley M, Zola B. Urokinase plus heparin versus aspirin in unstable angina and non-Q-wave myocardial infarction. Am J Cardiol 1989; 64: 840–844.
7. Olson HG, Lyons KP, Aronow WS, Stinson PJ, Kuperus J, Waters HJ. The high-risk angina patient. Identification by clinical features, hospital course, electrocardiography and technetium-99 m stannous pyrophosphate scintigraphy. Circulation 1981; 64: 674–684.
8. Donsky MS, Curry GC, Parkey RW, Meyer SL, Bonte FJ, Platt MR, Willerson JT. Unstable angina pectoris. Clinical, angiographic and myocardial scintigraphic observations. Br Heart J 1976; 38: 257–263.
9. Jaffe AS, Klein MS, Patel BR, Siegel BA, Roberts R. Abnormal technetium-99 m pyrophosphate images in unstable angina: ischemia versus infarction? Am J Cardiol 1979 44: 1035–1039.
10. Poliner L, Buja LM, Parker RW, Bonte FJ, Willerson JT. Clinicopathologic findings in 52 patients studied by technetium-99 m stannaous -pyrophsphate myocardial scintigraphy. Circulation 1979; 59: 257–267.
11. Guthrie RB, Vlodaver Z, Nicoloff DM, Edwards J. Pathology of stable and unstable angina pectoris. Circulation 1975; 51: 1059–1063.
12. Fuster V, Badimon L, Badimon JJ, Chesebro JH. The pathogenesis of coronary artery disease and the acutre coronary syndromes. N Engl J Med 1992;326:242–250.
13. Scanlon PJ, Nemickas R, Moran JF, Talano JV, Amirpirviz F, Pifarre R. Accelerated angina pectoris: clinical, hemodynamic, arteriographic and therapeutic experience in 85 patients. Circulation 1973; 47: 19–27.
14. Ouyang P, Brinker JA, Mellits ED, Weisfeldt ML, Gerstenblith G. Variables predictive of successful medical therapy in patients with unstable angina: selection by multivariate analysis from clinical, electrocardiographic and angiographic evaluations. Circulation 1984; 70: 367–376.
15. Plotnick G, Conti CR. Unstable angina: angiography, morbidity and mortality of medically treated patients. Am J Med 1977; 63: 870–879.
16. Allison HV, Russell RO, Mantle JA, Kouchoukos N, Moraski RE, Rackley CE. Coronary anatomy and arteriography in patients with unstable angina pectoris. Am J Cardiol 1978; 204–209.
17. Fowler NO. "Pre-infarctional" angina. A need for an objective definition and for a controlled clinical trial of its management. Circulation 1971; 44:753–758.
18. Gazes PC, Mobley EM, Faris HM Jr, Duncan RC, Humphries GP. Preinfarction (unstable angina) - a prospective study - ten year follow-up. Prognostic significance of electrocardiographic changes. Circulation 1973; 48: 331–337.
19. Krauss KR, Hutter AM Jr, DeSanctis RW. Acute coronary insufficiency. Course and follow-up. Arch Intern Med 1972;129:808–813.

20. Fulton M, Duncan B, Lutz W, Morrison SL, Donald KW, Kerr F, Kirby BJ, Julian DG. Natural history of unstable angina. Lancet 1972;I:860–865.
21. Mulcahy R, Awadhi A, Buitleor M, Tobin G, Johnson H, Contoy R. Natural history and prognosis of unstable angina. Am Heart J 1985; 109: 753–758.
22. Russell RO Jr, Moraski RE, Kouchoukos N and the Unstable angina pectoris Study Group. Unstable angina pectoris: National Cooperative Study group to compare surgical and medical therapy. II. In-hospital experience and initial follow-up results in patients with one, two, and three vessel disease. Am J Cardiol 1978; 42: 839–848.
23. Duncan B, Fulton M, Morrison SL, Lutz W, Donald KW, Kerr F, Kirby BJ, Julian DG, Oliver MF. Prognosis of new and worsening angina pectoris. Br Med J 1976;1:981–985
24. Langer A, Freeman MR, Armstrong PW. ST segment shift in unstable angina: Pathophysiology and association with coronary anatomy and hospital outcome. J Am Coll Cardiol 1989; 13: 1495–1502.
25. Gottlieb SO, Weisfeldt MLK, Ouyang P, Mellits ED, Gerstenblith G. Silent ischemia as a marker for early unfavorable outcome in patients with unstable angina. N Engl J Med 1986; 314: 1214–1219.
26. Lewis HD, Davis JW, Archibald DG, Steinke WE, Smitherman TC, Doherty JE, Schnaper HW, LeWinter MM, Linares E, Pouget JM, Sabharwal SC, Chesler E, DeMots H. Protective effects of aspirin against acute myocardial infarction and death in men with unstable angina. N Engl J Med 1983;309:396–403.
27. Heng MK, Norris RM, Singh BN, Partridge JB. Prognosis in unstable angina. Br Heart J 1976; 38:921–925.
28. Mulcahy R, Daly L, Graham I, Hickey N, O'Donoghue S, Owens A, Ruane P, Tobin G. Unstable angina. Natural history and determinants of prognosis. Am J Cardiol 1981; 48:525–528.
29. Theroux P, Ouimet H, McCans J, Latour JG, Joly P, Levy G. Aspirin, heparin, or both to treat acute unstable angina. N Engl J Med 1988; 319:1105–1111.
30. Figueras J, Lidon RM. Coronary reserve, extent of coronary disease, recurrent angina and ECG changes during pain in the in-hospital prognosis of acute coronary syndromes. Eur Heart J 1993;14:185–194.
31. The Timi IIIb Investigators. Effects of Tissue plasminogen activator and a comparison of early invasive and conservative strategies in unstable angina and non-Q-wave myocardial infarction. Results of the TIMI IIIb trial. Circulation 1994;89;1545–1556.
32. Fragmin during instability in Coronary Artery Disease (FRISC) study group. Low-molecular-weight heparin during instability in coronary artery disease. Lancet 1996;347:561–568.
33. Figueras J, Cinca J, Valle V, Rius J. Prognostic implications of early spontaneous angina after acute transmural myocardial infarction. Int J Cardiol 1983;4:261–272.
34. Bugiardini R, Pozzati A, Borghi A, Morgagni JL, Ottani F, Muzi A, Puddu P. Angiographic morphology in unstable angina and its relation to transient myocardial ischemia and hospital outcome. Am J Cardiol 1991;67:460–464.
35. Bertolet BD, Dinerman J, Hartke R Jr, Conti CR. Unstable angina. Relationship of clinical presentation, coronary artery pathology, and clinical outcome. Clin Cardiol 1993;16:116–122.
36. The Global Use of Strategies to open occluded coronary arteries (GUSTOIIb) Investigators. A comparison of recombinant hirudin with heparin for the treatment of acute coronary syndromes. N Engl J Med 11996;335:775–782.
37. Sclarovsky S, Davidson E, Lewin RF, Strasberg B, Arditti A, Agmon J. Unstable angina pectoris evolving to acute myocardial infarction: significance of ECG changes during chest pain. Am Heart J 1986; 112: 459–462.
38. Holdright DR, Patel D, Cunningham D, Thomas R, Hubbard W, Hendry G, Sutton G, Fox K. Comparison of the effects of heparin and aspirin versus aspirin alone on transient myocardial ischemia and in-hospital prognosis in patients with unstable angina. J Am Coll Cardiol 1994;24:39–45.
39. Organization to assess strategies for ischemic syndromes (OASIS) investigators. Comparison of the effect of two doses of recombinant hirudin compared with heparin in patients with acute myocardial ischemia without ST elevation. Circulation 1997;96:769–777.

40. Klein W, Buchwald A, Hillis SE, Mionrad S, Sanz G, Turpie GG, Van der Meer J, Olaisson E, Undeland S, Ludwig K. For the FRIC investigators. Comparison of low-molecular-weight heparin with unfractionated heparin acutely and with placebo for 6 weeks in the management of unstable coronary artery disease. Fragmin in unstable coronary artery disease study (FRIC). Circulation1997;96:61-68.

41. Cohen M, Demers C, Gurfinkel E, Turpie A, Fromell GJ, Langer A, Califf RM, Fox KAA, Premmereur J, Bigonzi F (Essence) A comparison of low molecular weight heparin with un fractionated heparin for unstable coronary artery disease. Efficacy and safety of subcutaneous enoxaparine in non Q-wave coronary events Studty Group, N Engl Jmed 1997;337:447-452.

42. Balsano F, Rizzon P, Violi F, Scrutinio D, Cimminiello C, Aguglia F. Antiplatelet treatment with ticlopidine in unstable angina. A controlled multicenter clinical trial. Circulation 1990;82: 17-26.

43. Papapietro SE, Niess GS, Paine TD, Mantle JA, Rackley CE, Russell RO Jr, Rogers WJ. Transient electrocardiographic changes in patients with unstable angina: relation to coronary arterial anatomy. Am J Cardiol 1980; 46: 28-33.

44. DeServi S, Ghio S, Ferrario M, Ardissino D, Angoli L, Mussini A, Bramucci E, Salerno V, Vigano M, Montemartini C, Specchia G. Clinical and angiographic findings in angina at rest. Am Heart J 1986; 111: 6-11.

45. Plotnick GD. Unstable angina. A clinical approah. Futura Pub. Comp. Inco. New York, 1985,191-199.

46. Nadamanee K, Intarachit V, Josephson MA, Rieders D, Vaghaiwalla F, Singh BN. Prognostic significance of silent myocardial ischemia in patients with unstable angina. J Am Coll Cardiol 1987; 10: 1-9.

47. Armstrong PW, Chiong MA, Parker JO. The spectrum of unstable angina: Prognostic role of serum creatine kinase determination. Am J Cardiol 1982; 49: 1849-1852.

48. Hamm CW, Ravkilde J, Gerhaardt W, Jorgensen P, Peheim E, Ljungdahl L, Goldmann B, Katys HA. The prognostic value of serum troponin T in unstable angina. N EnglJ Med 1992:327;146-150.

49. Nixon JV, Hillert MC, Shapiro W, Smitherman T. Submaximal exercise testing after unstable angina. Am Heart J 1980; 99:772-778.

50. Butman SM, Olson HG, Gradin JM, Piters KM, Hullet M, Butman LK. Submaximal exercise testing after ustabilization of unstable angina pectoris. J Am Coll Cardiol 1984; 4:667-673.

51. Swahn E, Areskog M, Berglund U, Walfridsson H, Wallentin L. Predictive importance of clinical findings and a predischarge exercise test in patients with suspected unstable coronary artery disease. Am J Cardiol 1987; 59: 208-214.

52. Scott SM, Luchi RJ, Deupree RH. Veterans Administration Cooperative Study for treatment of patients with unstable angina. Results in patients with abnormal left ventricular function. Circulation 1988;78:supp I:I:113-121.

53. Nyman I, Wallentin L, Areskpog M, Areskog NH, Swahn E. RISC study group. Risk stratification by early exercise testing after an episode of unstable coronary artery disease. In J Cardiol 1993;39:131-142.

54. Marmur JD, Freeman MR, Laanger A, Armstrong PW. Prognosis in medically stabilized unstable angina. Early Holter ST-segment monitoring compared with predischarge thallium tomography. Ann Intern Med 1990;113:575-578.

55. Brown KA. Prognostic value of thallium-201 myocadrial perfusion imaging in patients with unstable angina who respond to medical treatment. J Am Coll Cardiol 1991;17:1053-1057.

56. Romeo F, Rosano GMC, Martuscelli E, Vaalente A, Reale A Unstable angina: role of silent ischemia and total ischemic time (silent plus painful ischemia), a 6 year follow-up. J Am Coll Cardiol 1992;19;1173-1179.

57. Patel DJ, Holdright DR, Knight CJ Mulcahy D, Thakrar B, Wright C, Sparrow J, Wicks M, Hubbard W, Thomas R, Sutton GC, Hendry G, Purcell H, Fox K. Early continuous ST segment monitoring in unstable angina: prognostic value additional to the clinical characteristics and the admission electrocardiogram. Heart 1996;75:222-228.

58. Bugiardini R, Borghi A, Pozzati A, Ruggeri A, Puddu P, Maseri A. Relation of severity of symptoms to transient myocartdial ischemia and prognosis in unstable angina. J Am Coll Cardiol 1995;25:597–604.
59. Holmvang L, Lüscher MS, Clemensen P, Thygesen K, Graande P,. Very early stratification using combined ECG and biochemical assessment in patients with unstable coronary artery disease (A thrombin inhibition in Myocardial ischemia (TRIM) substudy. Circulation 1998;98:2004–2009.
60. Bär FW, Raynaud P, Renkin JP, Vermeer F, De Zwaan C, Wellens HJJ. Coronary arteriographic findings do not predict clinical outcome in patients with unstable angina. J Am Coll Cardiol 1994;24:1453–1459.
61. Maise AS, Ahrve S, Gilpin E, Henning H, Goldberger AL, Collins D, LeWinter M, Ross J Jr. Prognosis after extension of myocardial infarction: the role of Q wave and non-Q-wave infarction. Circulation 1985; 71: 211–217.
62. Gibson RS, Beller GA, Gheorghiades M, Nygaard TW, Watson DD, Huey BL, Sayre SL, Kaiser DL. The prevalence and clinical significance of residual myocardial ischemia 2 weeks after uncomplicated non-Q-wave infarction: a prospective natural history study. Circulation 1986; 73: 1186–1198.
63. Stratman HG, Tamesis BR, Youni LT, Wittry MD, Amato M, Miller DD. Prognostic value of predischarge dipyridamole technetium 99 m sestamibi myocardial tomography in medically treated patients with unstable angina. Am Heart J 1995;130:734740.
64. Kent KM, Rosing DR, Ewels CJ, Lipson L, Bonow R, Epstein SE. Prognosis of asymptomatic or mildly symptomatic patients with coronary artery disease. Am J Cardiol 1982; 49: 1823–1830.
65. Weiner DA, Ryan TJ, McCabe CH, Chaitman BR, Sheffield LT, Ferguson JC, Fisher LD, Tristan F. Prognostic importance of a clinical profile and exercise test in medically treated patients with coronary artery disease. J Am Coll Cardiol 1984; 3: 772–779.
66. Zalewski A, Shi Y, Nardone D, Bravettee B, Weinstock P, Fischman D, Wilson P, Goldberg S, Levin DC, Bjornsson TD. Evidence for reduced fibrinolytic activity in unstable angina at rest. Clinical, biochemical, and angiographic correlates. Circulation 1991;83:1685–1691.
67. Munkvad S, Gram J, Jespersen J. A depression of active tissue plasminogen activator in plasma characterizes patients with unstable angina pectoris who develop myocardial infarction. Eur Heart J 1990;11:525–528.
68. Liuzzo G, Biasucci LM, Gallimore RJ, Grillo RL, Rebuzzi AG, Pepys MB, Maseri A. The prognostic value of C-reactive protein and serum amyloyd A protein in severe unstable angina. N Engl J Med 1994;331:417–24.
69. Morrow DA, Rifai N, Antman EM, Weiner DL, McCabe CH, Cannon CP, Braunwald E. C-Reactive protein is a potent predictor of mortality independently of and in combination with troponin T in acute coronary syndromes: A TIMI 11 substudy. J Am Coll Cardiol 1998; 31:1460–1465.

Assessment of Myocardial Viability

A. Flotats, I. Carrió

Introduction

The assessment of the distinct states of non-contractile myocardium in patients with coronary artery disease (CAD) and left ventricular (LV) dysfunction is clinically relevant, both prognostically and therapeutically [1–4]. Such dysfunction can be improved by restoring the perfusion in presence of chronic ischemia in the case of hibernating myocardium [5], or can improve spontaneously over time after an ischemic episode in the case of stunned myocardium [6]. Improvement will not occur if scarring has replaced the myocardial tissue.

Pathophysiologic paradigms have emerged that describe the relationships between myocardial perfusion, metabolism and LV function, leading to these concepts of stunning and hibernation. Our understanding of these concepts is constantly changing as new data emerge, and we have much to learn with regard to the complex physiology involved in the pathogenesis of LV dysfunction, its reversal, and its relationship to patient outcome.

Importance of Viability Assessment

Although the definition of viable myocardium has classically been limited to stunned and hibernating myocardium by defining it as regions expected to show improved contractility after the passage of time or revascularization, respectively, more properly, it should encompass all non-infarcted myocardium (stunned, hibernating, transiently ischemic and normal myocardium). This definition is closer to the literal meaning of the word "viable" and implicitly acknowledges that there can be compelling reasons to revascularize transiently ischemic myocardium (having normal function in between episodes of ischemia) despite the fact that it would not be expected to demonstrate improved resting function afterwards.

The issue of hibernating myocardium is important only in patients with CAD and impaired LV function being considered for coronary revascularization, as these procedures often entail an increased perioperative mortality in such patients [7, 8]. However, this is the same population that may ultimately benefit the most from revascularization [4]. Therefore, it is important to prospectively identify with a great degree of confidence which patients with potentially reversible LV dysfunction would truly benefit from surgical intervention with respect to a low perioperative mortality and enhanced long-term event-free survival rate. On the other hand, newer revascularization strategies, such as laser revascularization techniques and drugs to stimulate myocardial angiogenesis may increase the importance of identification of viable myocardium.

As CAD is the leading cause of heart failure in the majority of developed countries [9], myocardial viability assessment has important implications in the treatment of patients with congestive heart failure. The percentage of patients with CAD and LV dysfunction undergoing myocardial revascularization who subsequently demonstrate improvement in LV function varies among 25%–40% [3, 10].

The preliminary data suggest that among patients referred for transplantation, a significant minority are actually better candidates for revascularization. The cost of implications of avoiding cardiac transplantation in favor of revascularization are enormous, and non-invasive assessment to create a comprehensive base of information on which to base these decisions is necessary [4].

Methods of Viability Assessment

The ability to detect patients with CAD and potentially reversible LV dysfunction is problematic and often can be made only retrospectively after revascularization procedures. Nevertheless, this is not adequate in many high-risk patients with LV dysfunction, in whom the decision to proceed with revascularization may depend in large part upon whether the myocardium within the coronary territory to be revascularized is considered viable. Therefore, accurate diagnostic techniques are required to prospectively provide this information. These include evaluation of regional perfusion, cell membrane integrity and metabolism with nuclear techniques, contractile reserve using dobutamine echocardiography or magnetic resonance imaging (MRI), and microvascular integrity using contrast echocardiography or MRI. The extend of CAD determined by the number of major vessels with significant stenoses does not provide information pertaining to whether such stenotic vessels are predominantly supplying myocardial zones that are chronically hypoperfused and viable compared to zones that have substantial areas of myocardial scar. Indexes of regional wall motion, regional systolic wall thickening and regional coronary blood flow are helpful in identifying viable tissue if they are normal or near-normal. However, in patients with LV dysfunction arising from viable but hibernating myocardium, by definition the hibernating regions have blood flow, wall motion and wall thickening severely reduced or absent [5, 11]. For this reason radionuclide tracers that reflect intact cellular metabolic processes or cell membrane integrity have intrinsic advantages over indexes of function and blood flow. This chapter will principally review the applications of nuclear cardiac procedures for the assessment of myocardial viability.

Assessment of Metabolic Activity and Blood Flow

LV dysfunction that improves functionally after revascularization must have enough blood flow and metabolic activity to sustain myocyte viability. Hence, identification of these regions with the combined assessment of regional blood flow and metabolism is the most well-established means by which to assess viability [12–14]. The measurement of blood flow is principally based on positron emission tomography (PET) studies with radiotracers of blood flow, being the ^{13}N-labeled ammonia (^{13}NH$_3$) the most widely used [15]. To assess whether metabolic activity is present in severely hypoperfused and dysfunctional myocardium, the greatest experience and validation has been achieved in PET studies using ^{18}Fluorodeoxyglucose (FDG) [16–20].

During ischemia cardiac oxidative metabolism shifts from the oxidation of long free chain fatty acids to that of anaerobic glycolysis, contributing glucose up to 70% of the total energy production [21]. Thus, glucose utilization is augmented in segments that are hypoperfused and ischemic but still viable, and allows the myocyte to produce high energy phosphates in the status of reduced oxygen availability [21, 22]. This condition may be insufficient to preserve regional mechanical work but may be sufficient to maintain processes which are fundamental to cell viability. These metabolic pathways persist only if a critical level of blood flow is maintained [21]. Furthermore, blood flow must be sufficient to remove the metabolites of the glycolytic pathway [21, 22].

After intravenous administration, FDG traces the initial transport of glucose across the myocyte membrane and its subsequent hexokinase-mediated phosphorylation to FDG-6-phosphate. This compound is relatively impermeable to cell membranes, because the enzyme that catalyzes the reverse reaction, glucose-6-phosphatase, is absent or present in only negligible quantities. Therefore, the tracer becomes trapped in the myocardium and its persistent activity reflects regional rates of exogenous glucose utilization. In myocardial segments with irreversible injury, tissue glucose utilization declines linearly with blood flow. Several distinct perfusion-metabolism patterns can be observed in dysfunctional myocardium: (1) normal blood flow associated with homogeneous (normal) FDG uptake; (2) reduced blood flow associated with normal or increased FDG uptake (perfusion-metabolism mismatch); (3) proportional reduction in blood flow and FDG uptake (perfusion-metabolism match); and (4) reduced FDG uptake associated with preserved blood flow. Patterns 1 and 2 identify potentially reversible myocardial dysfunction (stunning and hibernation, respectively), whereas patterns 3 and 4 identify irreversible myocardial dysfunction [16–20].

Available data on prediction of functional recovery using this combined method demonstrates it to be an accurate clinical marker of myocardial viability, with positive predictive values in the range of 52% to 100% (mean 76%±12%) with negative predictive values in the range of 67% to 100% (mean 82%±14%) [16, 20]. Moreover, there is evidence that the extent and magnitude of metabolic-blood flow mismatch in a patient with LV dysfunction can be used to predict the magnitude of recovery in global LV function after revascularization [16, 17], which appears to translate into an improvement in prognosis. Recently published data suggest that myocardial revascularization in patients with perfusion-metabolism FDG mismatch significantly improves survival compared to the survival results during medical therapy [18, 19]. The improvement in LV function after revascularization, as predicted by perfusion-metabolism mismatch, is also associated with a significant improvement in symptoms of congestive heart failure [19].

PET appears to be the most accurate technique for prediction of recovery of LV function after coronary revascularization [16], but its limited availability and high cost preclude its broader use. Technological advances in gammacamera and collimator design have permitted the ability to image FDG with widely available single photon emission computed tomography (SPECT) technology, with good to excellent concordance between this technique and PET [23].

The study of flow/FDG relationships is only one approach for the assessment of myocardial metabolism in ischemic conditions. Metabolic perturbation may occur on a cellular level as a result of acute or chronic ischemia and not be detected by flow/FDG relationships. Therefore, other markers of myocardial metabolism have been developed. ^{11}C-acetate is converted into acetyl-CoA, which is incorporated in tricarboxylic acid cycle. Hence, dynamic PET studies of myocardial uptake of ^{11}C-acetate kinetics provide noninvasive measurement of regional myocardial oxygen consumption and mitochondrial oxidative flux [24]. Furthermore, myocardial blood flow may be quantified using the same tracer injection. ^{11}C-acetate imaging has been reported to provide greater accuracy than FDG imaging for prediction of viability [25]. FDG seems to have less diagnostic specificity because there may be myocytes capable to incorporate glucose without an improvement of contractility. ^{11}C-acetate uptake, on the contrary, would only identify myocytes with preserved oxidative flux. Additional PET methods for assessing myocardial viability include the use of ^{15}O-water to determine the amount of perfusable tissue within dysfunctional myocardial segments [26].

As in ischemic myocardium fatty acid oxidation is greatly suppressed in favor of glucose metabolism [21], the alteration of fatty acid oxidation is considered to be a sensitive marker of ischemia and myocardial damage. There are two groups of iodinated fatty acid compounds used in SPECT imaging, strain chain fatty acid and modified branched fatty acids [27]. The former compounds, such as ^{123}I-labeled iodophenyl pentadecanoic acid (IPPA) are generally metabolized via β-oxidation and released from the myocardium. Therefore fatty acid use can be directly assessed by the washout kinetics of the tracer, although rapid dynamic acquisition is required. The modified fatty acids compounds, such as 15-(p-iodophenyl)-3R,S-methyl pentadecanoid acid (BMIPP), were introduced on the basis of the concept of myocardial retention resulting from metabolic trapping, and in comparison to the strain chain compounds, its cellular activity can no longer identify reduced β-oxidation as a marker of ischemia, but is dependent on cytosolic levels of adenosine triphosphate, which are reduced under conditions of ischemia [28]. Therefore, imaging of these iodinated fatty acids in conjunction with perfusion is required to demonstrate perfusion-metabolism mismatch and thus to characterize fatty acid utilization. In ischemic myocardium, relatively decreased BMIPP uptake compared to regional perfusion (perfusion-metabolism mismatch) identifies the region as recoverable, and may be the result of increased back diffusion of the nonmetabolized tracer from the myocardium [29]. There are a number of reports showing that the perfusion-metabolism BMIPP mismatch correlates to the perfusion-metabolism FDG mismatch in patients with chronic CAD [30]. Perfusion-metabolism BMIPP mismatch has been reported to be a good predictor of improvement of dysynergic wall motion after successful revascularization, and that the magnitude of the mismatch closely relates to the degree of wall motion improvement [31]. However, there are a few data that examine the predictive value of the mismatch pattern for wall motion improvement in the setting of chronic CAD.

Assessment of Perfusion and Cell Membrane Integrity

Radiotracers used for viability assessment in this category include ^{201}Tl, ^{99m}Tc-sestamibi, ^{99m}Tc-tetrofosmin, [99m]TcN-NOET, and, for PET imaging, [82]Rb. Although each of these agents displays different kinetics, the concept that their uptake is related to myocardial perfusion and that some aspect of their kinetics is related to cell membrane integrity and thus to viability is common to each of them. The dual properties of such tracers enhance their utility, since with appropriate analysis, much information can be gained from a single scan. These conventional radionuclide tracers are widely available and relatively reliable for the assessment of myocardial viability as compared with positron emission tracers. In general, they have a high sensitivity but a relatively low specificity for prediction of LV functional recovery [32]. Thallium-201 is the most widely used SPECT agent for viability assessment. The most common protocols used are stress-redistribution-reinjection [33], and rest-redistribution [34] imaging. Stress-redistribution-reinjection ^{201}Tl imaging has demonstrated a high sensitivity (from 80% to 100%), but a relatively low specificity (<50% in all but one study) for prediction of recovery of LV regional contraction [32]. Patients with reversible defects in the redistribution images were excluded in some studies, which may lead to an underestimation of the accuracy of this imaging protocol. If the clinical issue to be addressed is the viability of a dysfunctional region and not the presence of inducible ischemia, the rest-redistribution ^{201}Tl imaging protocol provides information with a sensitivity of 44% to 100% and specificity of 31% to 92% for prediction of recovery of LV contraction after revascularization [32]. It also predicts improvement of global LV function after revascularization with reasonable accuracy [34], and identifies a high-risk patient group if medically treated [35]. The data with regard to sestamibi imaging for viability assessment are promising as well, with a sensitivity of 73% to 100% and specificity of 35% to 86% for prediction of recovery of LV contractility [32]. In general, positive and negative predictive values (ranges of 45% to 91% and 59% to 100%, respectively) are similar to that reported for ^{201}Tl imaging [36, 37]. Controversy remains concerning its utility in patients with severe LV dysfunction. These studies and others underscore the importance of quantitative analysis for sestamibi imaging. Newer technetium-based agents such as tetrofosmin and NOET have not been studied so extensively for purposes of viability assessment. Tetrofosmin appears to correlate well with ^{201}Tl imaging when quantitative analytical methods are used, and a concordance with ^{201}Tl of 90% has been reported [38, 39], being similar to the 93% concordance reported between ^{201}Tl and sestamibi data [37]. NOET promises the potential of combining the more favorable imaging characteristics of ^{99m}Tc with the more favorable kinetics of ^{201}Tl and may prove to be a useful viability marker in future studies [40, 41]. Rubidium-82, a PET perfusion tracer, is similar to ^{201}Tl and sometimes is used for viability assessment using quantitative analysis of [82]Rb washout [42].

Enhanced detection of viable myocardium by nitrate administration before injection of these tracers has largely been demonstrated [38, 39, 43–48]. Nitrates increase myocardial blood flow to hypoperfused myocardial regions by dilating the stenotic lumen, facilitating flow through collateral channels due to the relaxation of the epicardial vessels, and improving subendocardial perfusion as a result of LV preload and afterload reduction. Because the administration of nitrates is simple and inexpensive, He et al [49] propose in a recent editorial, that unless contraindicated, they should be administered when assessing myocardial viability using tracers of perfusion and cell membrane integrity.

Although these perfusion tracers have less ability to identify hibernating myocardium as compared with the combined use of FDG and blood flow imaging, their ability to identify a region as viable can still be helpful as far as there must be a critical level of blood flow for preserved metabolic activity in viable tissue [21]. A patient with a large area of myocardium supplied by a subtotally or totally occluded coronary artery is much more likely to benefit from revascularization when perfusion imaging shows significant uptake of the agent in the region compared to when there is none.

With the introduction of ECG-gated SPECT perfusion imaging, it is now feasible to assess simultaneously myocardial perfusion and function [50]. The ECG-gated SPECT method permits precise registration between regional perfusion and regional function, which is not feasible when SPECT is combined with other imaging modalities. Studies have demonstrated good correlation between other imaging modalities in relation to ventricular wall motion [50, 51]. Although it is known that areas of stunned or hibernating myocardium are frequently akinetic, in many patients in whom revascularization is being considered the demonstration of preserved ventricular function in the distribution of a fixed perfusion defect may indicate viable, salvageable myocardium. As preserved wall motion/thickening is an obvious sign of myocardial viability that may help to clarify the status of segments with equivocal or intermediate tracer uptake, several ECG-gated SPECT imaging protocols have been developed. However, if no motion or thickening is present, viability cannot be excluded since areas of stunned or hibernating myocardium may be akinetic or even dyskinetic with no evidence of thickening but recover function following successful revascularization. The potential advantage of ECG-gated SPECT to assess viability is its availability with conventional technology and tracers, with minimal modifications to protocols already in widespread clinical use. Several studies have demonstrated a role of combined perfusion and function for prediction of viability [50, 52]. Another direction of potential interest is the use of the end-diastolic image alone to more precisely assess tracer uptake in dysfunctional segments. On the basis of the concepts of partial volume effects and recovery coefficient, a dysfunctional territory with similar uptake to an area of preserved function may appear to have a "defect", or less tracer uptake, because of the absence of local thickening and of remote wall thickening. Quantitatively assessing tracer uptake in the frozen end-diastolic frame alone may obviate this effect and allow better assessment of true tracer uptake.

Assessment of Inotropic Reserve: Dobutamine Studies

Dobutamine administration to assess inotropic reserve in viable myocardium has also shown considerable promise in assessing myocardial viability, in keeping with the presence of residual inotropic reserve in stunned and/or hibernating myocardium that may be elicited through catecholamine stimulation, which can be imagined during echocardiography [53, 54] or MRI [55, 56]. To make this determination, both wall thickening and endocardial excursion should be analyzed. Of these two parameters, an increase in wall thickening is a more specific marker of viability. Unfortunately, with echocardiography, assessment of wall thickening is often difficult, and analyses often rely heavily on wall motion changes. Assessment of wall thickening with MRI is easier and more uniformly evaluable, making it possible to derive quantitative information in any segment of the myocardium [56].

Dobutamine echocardiography has shown an average 83% positive predictive value and 81% negative predictive value for prediction of functional recovery after revascularization in patients with chronic LV dysfunction [57].

It will be important to determine how well inotropic induced changes in regional function can be detected with quantitative ECG-gated SPECT methods. Although dobutamine is not the preferred stress with SPECT perfusion imaging because the degree of coronary hyperemia is not maximal and myocardial tracer uptake underestimates flow, most patients in whom viability assessment is important have severe CAD, and thus the stress of dobutamine may be sufficient to induce myocardial ischemia in territory of diseased vessels [58]. Moreover, as dobutamine can also be infused at a low dose, acquisition of the ECG-gated SPECT images during the infusion, may permit an assessment of changes in regional function [59].

Assessment of Perfusion and Microvascular Integrity:
Myocardial Contrast Echocardiography and MRI

Myocardial contrast echocardiography (MCE) uses intravenous injection of microbubbles of air/inert gas, performing echocardiographic ultrasound imaging during the transition of the microbubbles through the intravascular space of the myocardium. This technique provides an estimate of microvascular integrity and perfusion [60]. It is too early to make definitive statements regarding the ability of MCE for detecting myocardial viability accurately. One comparative study has shown similar results between ^{201}Tl and intracoronary MCE regarding the identification of hibernating myocardium [61]. Nevertheless, in contrast to the development of radionuclide perfusion agents, there seems to be a very significant influence, not only of the distinct MCE agents on performance, but also an important influence of the imaging acquisition technique, of which there are already a wide variety of permutations. Furthermore, published data suggest that significant territories of the myocardium (particularly the inferior and lateral walls), are not adequately visualized [60]. Additionally, most analyses assess the contrast data independently of wall motion, whereas clinical application will demand incremental value with the use of an agent that adds expense to the study.

MRI is still in early stages of development, but it could have an enormous potential in cardiac imaging. First, myocardial perfusion by MRI has been studied with ultrafast sequences during the passage of a paramagnetic contrast agent, intravenously infused, through the myocardium. Such an MRI technique has considerable potential, and it seems likely to prove superior to myocardial contrast echocardiography [62]. Second, the use of fat-suppressed breath-hold MRI has been reported to produce high-resolution, noninvasive coronary angiograms [63]. Third, magnetic resonance spectroscopy is starting to be used for the evaluation of cardiac metabolism, and thus for viability assessment. The use of endogenous chemical species in the understanding of cellular dysfunction is extremely attractive. However, magnetic resonance spectroscopy remains technically demanding [64].

Comparison Between Nuclear and Echocardiographic Techniques in the Assessment of Myocardial Viability

Predictive values for recovery of regional wall motion after revascularization for dobutamine echocardiography and metabolic PET imaging with FDG are equivalent [13, 57, 65]. Nevertheless, the available data suggest that more patients and more myocardial segments appear viable with PET than with dobutamine echocardiographic studies, indicating that there are regions of viable myocardium that are metabolically active but lack inotropic reserve. The regions with discordant findings between the two techniques tend to be those in which blood flow is reduced at rest and are presumably hibernating. Contrarily, there is an excellent agreement between the two techniques in identifying dysfunctional myocardial regions that have preserved blood flow at rest and are presumably stunned [65]. These data would predict that dobutamine echocardiography would underestimate the potential for recovery of LV function in patients with CAD, and preliminary data obtained in patients before and after revascularization indicate that this appears to be the case [3].

Similar findings have been reported in the studies based on ^{201}Tl imaging. The level of ^{201}Tl activity can be used to predict the likelihood that a dysfunctional myocardial segment will manifest contractile reserve with dobutamine [57]. However, overall results suggest that dobutamine echocardiography has a higher specificity and a positive predictive value, but that ^{201}Tl SPECT imaging has a higher sensitivity and a negative predictive value [3, 57]. This higher specificity of dobutamine echocardiography can be explained in part on the basis of the "biphasic response" being an indicator not only of viability but also of inducible ischemia. Recently it has been reported that asynergic regions with reversible ^{201}Tl defects (inducible ischemia) on the pre-revascularization studies are more likely to improve after revascularization when compared with asynergic regions with mild-to-moderate fixed defects (79% vs. 30%, respectively, p<0.001) [66]. Even at a similar mass of viable myocardial tissue (as reflected by the final ^{201}Tl content), the presence of inducible ischemia is associated with an increased likelihood of functional recovery. Thus a more precise noninvasive determination of myocardial viability may require the demonstration of myocardial ischemia, which may explain the apparent suboptimal specificity of ^{201}Tl studies. Although preserved metabolic activity can be demonstrated in such segments, they may have only a moderate probability of functional recovery.

There are other possible explanations for this apparently lower specificity of nuclear studies in detecting myocardial viability, that is, why the detection of viable cells may not translate into a substantial recovery of regional function [3, 67]. First, it has to be well established the adequacy of revascularization. Second, the presence of only certain amount of tracer uptake in some territories at rest may represent the admixture of normally perfused and necrotic myocardium resulting from nontransmural necrosis. In such cases revascularization is not expected to affect regional function, although it may prevent inducible ischemia, LV dilation and remodeling, and reduce the risks of subsequent fatal cardiac events. Similarly, if there is an admixture of hypoperfused subepicardial myocardium and of necrotic subendocardial myocardium, revascularization would have no effect on recovery of function because of the lack of contribution of the subepicardium to regional systolic contraction. Third, irreversible ultrastructural changes in long-standing hibernation, including apoptosis, may also explain persistence of tracer uptake in irreversibly dysfunctional territories. Finally, there is a patient selection bias. It is possible that patients with evidence of predominant nonviable myocardium will less likely be referred for revascularization, and thus a large population of "true-negative" segments will not be included in the analysis of specificity.

The strengths of echocardiography in general are its availability and its relatively low cost. In addition to myocardial viability, the technique also permits anatomic assessment useful for decision making, such as cavity size, global left and right ventricular function, the level of LV pressures, the presence and severity of pulmonary hypertension, and valvular function. The weaknesses of echocardiography include poor acoustic windows in 10% to 20% of patients (due to obesity and pulmonary disease), making it difficult to assess wall motion and thickening in every LV segment. Several reports suggest that there is inadequate visualization of all myocardial segments in 37% of patients [57]. The recent introduction of second harmonic imaging may provide a better means of delineation of endocardial contours. The echocardiographic technique is operator dependent and thus requires a learning curve for both data acquisition and interpretation. This brings with it more interobserver and intraobserver variability than with nuclear techniques.

Conclusions

Comprehensive evaluation of patients with heart failure and LV systolic dysfunction should include an assessment of the underlying etiology (CAD or non-CAD causes), and if CAD is determined to be the etiology of the heart failure syndrome, an assessment of the potential for reversible LV dysfunction following revascularization (Fig. 1). This is related to the extent of inducible ischemia and preserved viability within dysfunctional myocardium. Thus, the assessment of myocardial viability (and often ischemia as well) is a clinically relevant issue in the setting of impaired global LV function, and in selected cases of isolated regional dysfunction if revascularization is contemplated. If function is preserved, it is obvious that viability is present; inducible ischemia then becomes the relevant issue. In properly selected patients, revascularization may result in improved symptoms, quality of life, exertional tolerance, ventricular function and perhaps survival. Even in the absence of an improvement in resting systolic regional or global performance, revascularization may favorably impact on several factors such as reduction of inducible ischemia, prevention of myocardial infarction and further remodeling, improvement in the arrhythmia milieu, improvement in diastolic function, and improvement in contractile reserve.

The ability of nuclear cardiology to distinguish myocardial viability on the basis of metabolic activity, perfusion and cell membrane integrity provides greater precision than that achieved by assessment of regional anatomy or function. Numerous scintigraphic techniques have been used for this purpose, and some general principles emerging from the literature can be summarized as follows:

1. In dysfunctional myocardial regions, the demonstration of inducible ischemia in stress and rest imaging, or rest ischemia by a "mismatch" in PET imaging, is a powerful predictor of functional recovery after revascularization.

2. The response of global LV function to revascularization is dependent on the number of ischemic but viable territories that are successfully revascularized; thus, the patients who will benefit most are those with the most extensive ischemic viable myocardium.

3. Isotope content itself within a dysfunctional territory is related to the mass of viable tissue and correlates with metabolic activity and the probably of func-

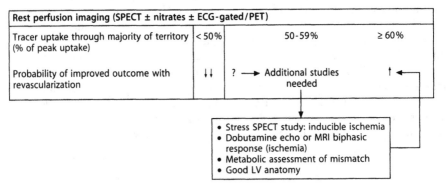

Fig. 1. Proposed clinical approach in patients with CAD and LV dysfunction

tional recovery. However, functional recovery is dependent on the presence of a sufficient mass of viable tissue to support regional contractile activity. For optimizing outcomes and reducing costs, revascularization strategies might be directed predominantly to patients with CAD who have coronary vessels suitable for revascularization and a noninvasive assessment of viability showing that ≥40%–50% of dysfunctional myocardium exhibits viability.

4. "Fixed" or "reversible" defects in SPECT perfusion imaging are incomplete descriptors for the purposes of assessing ischemia and viability in LV dysfunction: the magnitude of reversibility as well as the isotope content within the fixed defects are important correlates of regional myocardial viability. Even though the presence of ≥50% of isotope uptake in dysfunctional regions may have a suboptimal positive predictive value for predicting improved segmental function after revascularization, it appears to predict a high cardiac death and infarction rate with medical therapy.

5. Evidence of extensive ischemic viable in the setting of LV dysfunction (by anyone of several imaging techniques) is associated with a high risk of adverse cardiac events in the absence of revascularization.

A promising role for the metabolic agents will be in sorting out those patients with combined disease processes, for instance, a patient with a hypertensive or valvular cardiomyopathy who also has CAD. By demonstrating abnormal metabolism, these agents will probably be much more accurate than perfusion and cell membrane integrity agents in identifying those patients most likely to benefit from revascularization.

Despite the preponderance of literature in which improvement in LV function is a clinical end point, the real purpose of revascularization is to improve patient outcome, as assessed by morbidity and mortality. Thus, although the available information suggests that viability assessment may be prognostically important, there are unresolved issues regarding the knowledge of the pathophysiologic components of LV dysfunction in CAD an how this could be applied to clinical processes. Additional large scale studies are needed to confirm that such assessment is important in selecting patients for revascularization. It would be important to assess if revascularization is beneficial to clinical outcome even in the absence of improvement in LV function and/or in the absence of viable myocardium. At the current time, the identification of viable myocardium is not in and of itself an indication for revascularization, and the likelihood of recovery of myocardial dysfunction is also related to other factors, such as the degree of LV remodeling. Hence, as in any other patient with CAD, the decision to revascularize should be based on clinical presentation, coronary anatomy, LV function, LV geometry, and evidence of inducible ischemia. The knowledge that a large region of the LV is viable rather than irreversibly damaged will aid in this decision-making process, but it should not be the primary indication for revascularization.

References

1. Bonow RO, Epstein SE. Indications for coronary artery bypass surgery: implications of the multicenter randomized trials. Circulation 1982; 66: 562–568
2. Iskandrian AS, Heo J, Stanberry C. When is myocardial viability an important clinical issue?. J Nucl Med 1994; 35 (Suppl): 4S-7 S
3. Bonow RO. Identification of viable myocardium. Circulation 1996; 94: 2674–2680
4. Beller GA. Selecting patients with ischemic cardiomyopathy for medical treatment, revascularization, or heart transplantation. J Nucl Cardiol 1997; 4 (suppl):S152–77
5. Rahimtoola SH. The hibernating myocardium. Am Heart J 1989;117: 211–213
6. Braunwald E, Kloner RA. The stunned myocardium: prolonged, postischemic ventricular dysfunction. Circulation 1982; 66: 1146–1149
7. Kennedy JW, Kaiser GC, Fisher LD, et al. Clinical and angiographic predictors of operative mortality from the collaborative study in coronary artery surgery (CASS). Circulation 1981; 63: 793–802
8. Warner CD, Weintraub WS, Craver JM, Jones WL, Gott JP, Guyton RA. Effect of cardiac surgery patient characteristics on patient outcomes from 1981 through 1995. Circulation 1997; 96: 1575–1579
9. Kannel WB. Epidemiologic aspects of heart failure. Cardiol Clin 1989; 7: 1–9
10. Dilsizian V, Bonow RO, Cannon RO, et al. The effect of coronary artery bypass grafting on left ventricular systolic function at rest: evidence for preoperative subclinical myocardial ischemia. Am J Cardiol 1988; 61: 1248–1254
11. Dilsizian V, Bonow RO. Current diagnostic techniques of assessing myocardial viability in patients with hibernating and stunned myocardium. Circulation 1993; 87: 1–20
12. Tamaki N. Current status of viability assessment with positron tomography. J Nucl Cardiol 1994; 1: 40–47
13. Schelbert HR. Merits and limitations of radionuclide approaches to viability and future developments. J Nucl Cardiol 1994; 1 (Suppl): S86-S96
14. Bergmann SR. Use and limitations of metabolic tracers labeled with positron-emiting radionuclides in the identification of viable myocardium. J Nucl Med 1994; 35 (Suppl); 15–22
15. Schelbert HR, Phelps ME, Huang SC, et al. Nitrogen-13 ammonia as an indicator of myocardial blood flow. Circulation 1981; 63: 1259–1272
16. Tillisch JH, Brunken R, Marsahll R, et al. Reversibility of cardiac wall-motion abnormalities predicted by positron tomography. N Engl J Med 1986; 314: 884–888
17. Nienaber CA, Brunken RC, Sherman CT, et al. Metabolic and functional recovery of ischemic human myocardium after coronary angioplasty. J Am Coll Cardiol 1991; 18: 966–978
18. Eitzman D, Al-Aouar Z, Kanter HL, et al. Clinical outcome of patients with advanced coronary artery disease after viability studies with positron emission tomography. J Am Coll Cardiol 1992; 20: 569–565
19. Di Carli MF, Davidson M, Little R, et al. Value of metabolic imaging with positron emission tomography for evaluating prognosis in patients with coronary artery disease and left ventricular dysfunction. Am J Cardiol 1994; 73: 527–533
20. Tamaki N, Kawamoto M, Tamadura E, et al. Prediction of reversible ischemia after revascularization: perfusion and metabolic studies with positron emission tomography. Circulation 1995; 91:1694–1705
21. Camici P, Ferrannini E, Opie LH. Myocardial metabolism in ischemic heart disease: basic principles and application to imaging by positron emission tomography. Prog Cardiovasc Dis 1989; 32: 217–238
22. Opie LH. Effects of regional ischemia on metabolism of glucose and fatty acids: relative rates of aerobic and anaerobic energy production during myocardial infarction and comparison with effects of anoxia. Circ Res 1976; 38 (Suppl I): I-72-I-74

23. Bax JJ, Cornel JH, Visser FC, et al. Prediction of recovery of left ventricular dysfunction following revascularization: comparison F-18 Fluorodeoxyglucose SPECT, thallium stress-reinjection SPECT and dobutamine echocardiography. J Am Coll Cardiol 1996; 28:558–564

24. Gropler RJ, Geltman EM, Sampathkumaran K, et al. Functional recovery after coronary revascularization for chronic coronary artery disease is dependent of maintenance of oxidative metabolism. J Am Coll Cardiol 1992; 20: 569–577

25. Gropler RJ, Geltman EM, Sampathkumaran K, et al. Comparison of carbon-11-acetate with fluorine-18-fluorodiocyglucose for delineating viable myocardium by positron emission tomography. J Am Coll Cardiol 1993; 23: 1587–1597

26. de Silva R, Yamamoto Y, Rhodes CG, et al. Preoperative prediction of the outcome of coronary revascularization using positron emission tomography. Circulation 1992; 86: 1738–1742

27. Tamaki N, Fujibayashi Y, Magata Y, et al. Radionuclide assessment of myocardial fatty acid metabolism by PET and SPECT. J Nucl Cardiol 1995; 2: 256–266

28. Fujibayashi Y, Yonekura Y, Takemura Y, et al. Myocardial accumulation of iodinated beta-methyl-branched fatty acid analogue, iodine-125-15 (p-iodophenyl)-3-(R,S)methylpentadecanoic acid (BMIPP), in relation to ATP concentration. J Nucl Med 1990; 31: 1818–1822

29. Hosokawa R, Nohara R, Fujibayashi Y, et al. Myocardial kinetics of iodine-123-BMIPP in canine myocardium after regional ischemic and reperfusion: implications for clinical SPECT. J Nucl Med 1997; 38: 1857–1863

30. Tamaki N, Tamadura E, Kawamoto M, et al. Decreased uptake of iodinated branched fatty acid analog indicates metabolic alterations in ischemic myocardium. J Nucl Med 1995; 36: 1974–1980

31. Franken PR, Dendale P, DeGeeter F, et al. Prediction of functional outcome after myocardial infarction using BMIPP and sestamibi scintigraphy. J Nucl Med 1996; 37: 718–722

32. Bax JJ, Wijns W, Cornel JH, Visser FC, Boersma E, Fioretti PM. Accuracy of currently available techniques for prediction of functional recovery after revascularization in patients with left ventricular dysfunction due to chronic coronary artery disease: comparison of pooled data. J Am Coll Cardiol 1997; 30: 1451–1460

33. Dilsizian V, Rocco TP, Freedman NM, Leon MB, Bonow RO. Enhanced detection of ischemic but viable myocardium by the reinjection of thallium after stress-redistribution imaging. N Engl J Med 1990; 323: 141–146

34. Iskandrian AS, Hakki AH, Kane SA, Goel IP, Mundth ED, Segal BL. Rest and redistribution thallium-201 myocardial scintigraphy to predict improvement in left ventricular function after coronary arterial bypass grafting. Am J Cardiol 1983; 51: 1312–1315

35. Gioia G, Powers J, Heo J, Iskandrian AS. Prognostic value of rest-redistribution tomographic thallium-201 imaging in ischemic cardiomyopathy. Am J Cardiol 1995; 75: 759–762

36. Udelson JE, Coleman PS, Matherall JA, et al. Predicting recovery of severe regional ventricular dysfunction: comparison of resting scintigraphy with thallium-201 and technetium-99 m sestamibi. Circulation 1994; 89: 2552–2561

37. Dilsizian V, Arrighi JA, Diodati JG, et al. Myocardial viability in patients with chronic coronary artery disease. Comparison of ^{99m}Tc-sestamibi with thallium reinjection and [18F]Fluorodeoxyglucose. Circulation 1994; 89: 578–587

38. Matsunari I, Fulino S, Taki J, et al. Myocardial viability assessment with technetium-99m-tetrofosmin and thallium-201 reinjection in coronary artery disease. J Nucl Med 1995; 36: 1961–1967

39. Flotats A, Carrió I, Estorch M, et al. Nitrate administration to enhance the detection of myocardial viability by technetium-99 m tetrofosmin single-photon emission tomography. Eur J Nucl Med 1997; 24: 767–773

40. Ghezzi C, Fagret D, Arvieux CC, et al. Myocardial kinetics of 99mTcN-NOET: a neutral lipophilic complex tracer of regional myocardial blood flow. J Nucl Med 1995; 336: 1069–1073

41. Vanzetto G, Calnon D, Ruiz M, et al. Myocardial uptake and redistribution of 99mTcN-NOET in dogs with either sustained coronary low flow or transient coronary occlusion. Circulation 1997; 96: 2325-2331

42. Vom Dahl J, Muzik O, Wolfe ER, Alllman C, Hutchins G, Schwaiger M. Myocardial rubidium-82 tissue kinetics assessed by dynamic positron emission tomography as a marker of myocardial cell membrane integrity and viability. Circulation 1996; 93: 238-245

43. He ZX, Darcourt J, Guignier A, et al. Nitrates improve detection of ischemic but viable myocardium by thallium-201 reinjection SPECT. J Nucl Med 1993; 34: 1472-1477

44. Bisi G, Sciagrà R, Santoro GM, Rossi V, Fazzini PF. Technetium-99m-sestamibi imaging with nitrate infusion to detect viable hibernating myocardium and predict recovery. J Nucl Med 1995; 36: 1994-2000

45. He ZX, Verani MS, Liu XJ. Nitrate-augmented myocardial imaging for assessment of myocardial viability. J Nucl Cardiol 1995; 2: 352-357

46. Maurea S, Cuocolo A, Soricelli A, et al. Enhanced detection of viable myocardium by technetium-99m-MIBI imaging after nitrate administration in chronic coronary artery disease. J Nucl Med 1995; 36: 1945-1952

47. Sciagrà R, Bisi G, Santoro GM, Agnolucci M, Zoccarato O, Fazzini PF. Influence of the assessment of defect severity and intravenous nitrate administration during tracer injection on the detection of viable hibernating myocardium with data-based quantitative technetium 99m-labeled sestamibi single-photon emission computed tomography. J Nucl Cardiol 1996; 3: 221-230

48. Flotats A, Carrió I, Estorch M, et al. Valoración de la viabilidad miocárdica mediante SPET cardíaco de perfusión. Talio-201 reposo/redistribución, talio-201 reposo/reinyección y tecnecio 99m-tetrofosmina reposo-postnitratos. Rev Esp Cardiol 1998; 51 (Supl 1): 45-56

49. He ZX, Verani MS. Evaluation of myocardial viability by myocardial perfusion imaging: should nitrates be used?. J Nucl Cardiol 1998; 5: 527-532

50. Chua T, Kiat H. Germano G, et al. Gated technetium-99 m sestamibi for simultaneous assessment of stress myocardial perfusion, postexercise regional ventricular function and myocardial viability: correlation with echocardiography and rest thallium-201 scintigraphy. J Am Coll Cardiol 1994; 23: 1107-1114

51. Williams KA, Taillon LA. Left ventricular function in patients with coronary artery disease assessed by gated tomographic myocardial perfusion images: comparison with assessment by contrast ventriculography and first-pass radionuclide angiography. J Am Coll Cardiol 1996; 27: 173-181

52. Levine MG, McGill CC, Ahlberg AW, et al. Functional assessment with electrocardiographic gated single-photon emission computed tomography improves the ability of technetium-99 m sestamibi myocardial perfusion imaging to predict myocardial viability in patients undergoing revascularization. Am J Cardiol 1999; 83: 1-5

53. Afridi I, Kleinman NS, Raizner AE, Zoghbi WA. Dobutamine echocardiography in myocardial hibernation: optimal dose and accuracy in predicting recovery of ventricular function after coronary revascularization. Circulation 1995; 91: 663-670

54. Chaudhry FA. The role of stress echocardiography versus stress perfusion: a view from the other side. J Nucl Cardiol 1996; 3: S66-S74

55. Baer FM, Voth E, Schneider CA, Theissen P, Schicha H, Sechtem U. Comparison of low dose dobutamine gradient echo magnetic resonance imaging and positron emission tomography with fluorodeoxyglucose in patients with chronic coronary artery disease: a functional and morphological approach to the detection of residual myocardial viability. Circulation 1995; 91: 1006-1015

56. Gesken G, Kramer CM, Rogers W, et al. Quantitative assessment of myocardial viability after infarction by dobutamine magnetic resonance imaging. Circulation 1998; 98: 217-223

57. Bonow RO. Diagnosis and risk stratification in coronary artery disease: nuclear cardiology versus stress echocardiography. J Nucl Cardiol 1997; 4: S172-S178

58. Calnon DA, Glover DK, Beller GA, et al. Effects of dobutamine stress on myocardial blood flow, Tc-99 m sestamibi uptake and systolic wall thickening in the presence of coronary artery stenosis. Implications for dobutamine stress testing. Circulation 1997; 96: 2553–2560

59. Iskandrian AE, Acio E. Methodology of a novel myocardial viability protocol. J Nucl Cardiol 1998; 5: 206–209

60. Kaul S. Myocardial contrast echocardiography in coronary artery disease: potential applications using venous injection of contrast. Am J Cardiol 1995; 75: 61D-68D

61. Nagueh SF, Vaduanathan P, Ali N, et al. Identification of hibernating myocardium: comparative accuracy of myocardial contrast echocardiography, rest-redistribution thallium-201 tomography and dobutamine echocardiography. J Am Coll Cardiol 1997; 29: 985–993

62. Blackwell GG, Pohost GM. The evolving role of MRI in the assessment of coronary artery disease. Am J Cardiol 1995; 75: 74D-78D

63. Manning WJ, Li W, Edelman RR. A preliminary report comparing magnetic resonance coronary angiography with conventional angiography. N Engl J Med 1993; 328: 823–832

64. De Roos A, Van der Wall EE. Magnetic resonance imaging and spectroscopy of the heart. Curr Opin Cardiol 1991: 6: 946–952

65. Sawada S, Elsner G, Segar DS, et al. Evaluation of patterns of perfusion and metabolism in dobutamine-responsive myocardium. J Am Coll Cardiol 1997; 29: 55–61

66. Kitsiou AN, Srinivasan G, Quyyumi AA, Summers RM, Bacharach SL, Dilsizian V. Stress-induced reversible and mild-to-moderate irreversible thallium defects: are they equally accurate for predicting recovery of regional left ventricular function after revascularization?. Circulation 1998; 98: 501–508

67. Castell Conesa J, González González JM. Diagnóstico isotópico del miocardio viable. In: Candell J, Castell J, Aguadé J, editors. Miocardio en riesgo y miocardio viable. Diagnóstico mediante SPET. Barcelona: Ediciones Doyma, S.A., 1998; 203–236

Functional Assessment of the Coronary Physiology: The Role of Magnetic Resonance

J.F. Toussaint

Introduction

Nuclear Magnetic Resonance has recently emerged in cardiac physiology and cardiology. The absence of radiation exposure, the capability of imaging the entire heart volume, the development of fast imaging methods that can be performed on conventional MR systems are some of the several advantages, that have made MRI a reference imaging technique for evaluation of cardiac and coronary physiology. The MR signal depends on multiple parameters that all together represent the various aspects of cardiac metabolisms and functions: chemical composition, molecular motion, diffusion, physical state, water and lipid content, fiber orientation, perfusion, flow velocity. Fast MR imaging sequences use this dependence in order to assess: coronary anatomy (MR coronarography) and flow reserve (velocity by phase gradient encoding or time-of-flight), coronary wall imaging (spiral gradients), microcirculation (perfusion with endogenous or exogenous contrast agents), fiber orientation (diffusion) and contractility (tagging), high-energy phosphate metabolism, oxygen consumption and viability (by 31-Phosphorus or myoglobin spectroscopy), or global ventricular function. Spatial and temporal resolutions have considerably increased: images can now be acquired in less than 50 ms with a submillimetric matrix (Fig. 1). Also, the aforementioned parameters can be evaluated at rest and under physiological or pharmacological stress, and combined in a single comprehensive examination. This evaluation has the potential of aiding physicians in their therapeutic decisions eg coronary revascularization and helping them to plan and follow measures of primary or secondary prevention. Respecting the usual contraindications [1], MRI is safe and applicable even in the acute phase of a myocardial infarction. Echoplanar, Turboflash and Spiral interactive realtime imaging are the major methods which make this technology a major instrument of clinical and basic research in coronary physiology.

Anatomy: MR Angiography and Tissue Characterization

X-ray angiography is currently the first evaluation method for assessing coronary anatomy. It enables the determination of the extent of atherosclerotic disease, and guides therapy which may be performed during angiography. In the recent years, MR coronary angiography has largely progressed to overcome its previous limitations: resolution, the difficulty to acquire 3-dimensional datasets, and the need for long breathholding periods [2].

MR angiography takes advantage of the effect of saturation to reduce signal from structures in an imaging slice with bright signal generated by blood flowing into the imaging slice, thereby producing luminal images. This method is well suited to rapid imaging techniques which can be applied during a breath hold, an important feature for a complex moving target (heart and lung motions interfere with the necessity of always acquiring the same volume of data). This latter approach has been applied by several groups to generate coronary MR angiograms [3–8]. Two other approaches have been applied to clinical evaluation. The segmented k-space method uses a breathhold during acquisition to generate single slices. Manning et al. have shown that vessel diameter by this method correlates closely with similar measurements by X-ray contrast angiography. Other groups have investigated a full 3D acquisition approach for coronary imaging [9–10]. This area will receive much additional investigation in the close future, as it will play an important role in all types of non invasive coronary evaluation.

Tissue characterization of atheromatous plaques may have an impact on diagnosis and prognosis, for it may help to predict plaque rupture in coronary arteries. In vitro examinations of human specimens have demonstrated discrimination

Fig. 1. Real-time Echo-planar imaging allows the instant description of cardiac cycle at a rate of 10 images per heart beat. Spiral k-space acquisition may further enhance this speed

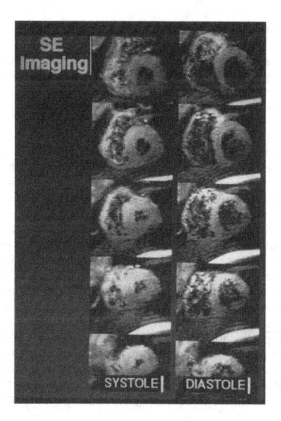

of plaque collagenous cap and lipid core in aortic, carotid, femoral and coronary arteries, and the characterization of lipid content [11]. The first in vivo studies have shown similar contrast in human carotid plaques in situ [12]. These data could allow the discrimination of stable from unstable lesions, and may help the surgical, medical or interventional decision. The first wall images of the circumflex coronary artery in the auriculoventricular groove using spiral acquisitions and fat saturation were recently produced, paving the way for a true non invasive approach to characterize both the impact of a lesion on hemodynamics and its potential for rupture [13]. Fayad et al. confirmed these results and showed that MRI provided an excellent description of lipid atheromatous cores in the coronaries [14].

Anomalous Coronary Arteries

Abnormal coronary vessels and ostia have been perfectly delineated by MR angiography using fast spin-echo [15] or more recently breathholded gradient-echo sequences [16]. The latter technique proved a better sensitivity and specificity than X-ray angiography for diagnosing the proximal course of these congenitaly abnormal vessels with a perfect interobserver agreement [17].

Flow Velocity Measurements

Assessment of coronary flow and flow reserve (CFR) uses two MR methods: one is based on phase velocity contrast, which takes advantage of the complex data (phase and magnitude) and the proportionality of phase shift of flowing spins to velocity in a magnetic field gradient (assuming constant velocity). The second option is the time-of-flight method: it is based on saturation, which causes signal to be reduced if stimulation pulses are applied too frequently (delay between radiofrequency stimulation less than 5 times the blood T1). Blood that flows into the slice has not been previously stimulated, and therefore produces an increase in signal intensity (refreshment) that is proportional to the amount flowing into the image since the last pulse. The ability to choose a variety of oblique planes permits an exact orthogonality with the main vessel lumen and ensures an accurate determination of flow velocity, which is not operator-dependent and can be automatically calculated. Coronary flow reserve is determined as usual by measurements at rest and in the presence of physiologic or pharmacologic vasodilatory stimuli. Several investigators have now applied the phase contrast technique to coronary velocity measurement. In one of these studies the investigators examined coronary flow velocity in normal subjects, demonstrating a flow reserve of approximately 5 in response to adenosine infusion [18]. The time of flight method was applied to the evaluation of coronary physiology by Poncelet et al. [19]. They used a rapid image acquisition technique, called echo planar imaging, which enables entire image acquisition in approximately 30 ms. Using this imaging method, heart motion can be frozen, thereby limiting coronary motion associated with slight variation in cardiac cycle or with patient movement (which could displace the coronary enough to corrupt the entire measurement). Observation of the refreshment of blood during the imaging sequence is enhanced by applying a presaturation pulse in the imaging plane to make the blood signal dark, and then image the coronary after an appropriate delay time. The investigators model this refreshment for multiple delay periods, using the model of parabolic flow. Using this method they are able to acquire images of gradual flow refreshment and calculate coronary flow velocity during various portions of the cardiac cycle, demonstrating its diastolic predominance. A study done with isometric exercise in the magnet showed a modest increase in flow velocity as a result of exercise, but because of the limited ability to perform exercise under the confined conditions of the magnet, it seems easier to use pharmacologic flow stimulation with dipyridamole. In such a study, CFR was approximately 4.5 in the normal subjects. In patients examined using the same protocol, with a 70% LAD stenosis, CFR was inferior to 2. This method is just beginning to be applied to a broad spectrum of patients with coronary disease, and it appears to hold great promise for a truly non-invasive evaluation of coronary physiology.

Coronary Microcirculation and Perfusion Assessment

Extrinsic Contrast Agents in First-Pass Studies

First-pass studies of Gadolinium-DTPA (FPMRI) relate to perfusion, and benefit from ultrafast imaging methods. The variable distribution of contrast agent between intra- and extra-vascular spaces does not yield a simple relation between signal enhancement and the concentration of administered Gd-DTPA making accurate perfusion measurement difficult. Also the uneven perfusion resulting from physiological heterogeneities of regional volumes of distribution and flows [20] and degree of collaterallization in CAD may make application of animal models of acute ischemia to human studies problematic. Despite these problems there have been several studies using the first-pass technique which have given optimistic results based on the calculation of perfusion indexes and more recently on true perfusion measurements. On a canine model, Wilke et al. demonstrated a good correlation between microsphere determined blood flow and the initial slope of the myocardial MR signal intensity curve [21]. The first-pass method has been applied to humans with encouraging results in normal subjects and patients with coronary artery disease. Early works comparing FPMRI to Positron Emission Tomography (PET) provide excellent agreement between these techniques with a sensitivity and specificity of nearly 90% [22] with the advantage of a higher resolution for MR allowing the determination of endocardial vs epicardial flow. In these studies, when compared to single photon nuclear scintigraphy with 201-Thallium or 99m-Technetium, FPMRI provides a higher sensitivity (92% vs. 85%) and a similar specificity (80%): this might be due to the fact that MR can discriminate a 20% flow reduction whereas a 30–40% reduction is required for accurate detection by scintigraphy. Therefore detection of mild flow reduction, of regional heterogeneities in multivessel diseases (a well-known and problematic false negative of scintigraphy that may occur in 5–10% of the cases, and the absence of radioactivity may non doubtly favor MRI in future large scale studies of myocardial perfusion.

Newer Contrast Agents

Recently developped contrast agents may allow better assessment of perfusion parameters. These are based on a chelate of Gd-DTPA with albumine or polylysine, determining its purely intravascular properties. Recent studies on various animal models have shown their interest in the determination of myocardial blood volume [23].

Paramagnetic dysprosium (Dy) and superparamagnetic iron oxide may increase our ability to determine the extent of ischemic regions. This effect results from an increase in magnetic susceptibility, which reduces T2 (caused by diffusion through the local magnetic field gradients). Using Dy-DTPA as a bolus injection, a series of images obtained with an echo-planar sequence can show the time course of contrast transit through myocardium [24]. The effect of dipyridamole induced coronary vasodilation can be seen as an earlier fall in signal and a more pronounced effect, suggesting a possible use of these agents to measure transit time and perfusion.

Intrinsic Contrast Agents

BOLD Effect

The determination of perfusion changes through blood oxygenation sensitive MRI (the BOLD effect, principle of brain functional MRI) has been demonstrated by Niemi et al. [25]. The important point of this study was to simultaneously assess perfusion and coronary flow reserve: the 14% increase in T2w signal intensity during dipyridamole infusion paralleled a 5–6 fold increase of coronary flow velocity. However, the BOLD effect is not assessable during inotropic stimulation (such as dobutamine) [26], for the increase in oxygen consumption reduces venous oxygen content and compensate for the increase of inflowing oxygenated hemoglobin; this may limit its application for combined studies of function and perfusion.

T1 Model of Perfusion

Exact quantification of myocardial perfusion has not yet been achieved in vivo. However, the model developed by Detre, Koretsky et al. [27] based on the effect of inflowing spins on apparent T1 has been applied with success to animal hearts. Excellent agreement have been demonstrated between MR and flowmeter measurements, as it was previously shown in brain perfusion when compared to radioactive microspheres [28]. However, the small expected changes (in the order of a few percent) makes it more challenging for the application to in vivo beating hearts (Fig. 2). Also the dependence upon the compartmentalization model used, [29] the difficult determination of blood volume and the slow water exchange rate in myocardial capillaries [30] does not allow a direct application of the model as it was done in skeletal muscle [31].

MR Assessment of Perfusion Defects and Permeability Alteration in Coronary Diseases

Despite the difficulties in interpretation of perfusion studies, studies have shown success in infarct quantification. Ovize et al. showed good infarct size correlation with MR images using Gd-DOTA, especially 6 h after the onset of reperfusion [32]. Two other studies showed a good correlation between Gd-enhanced MR images and the bed at risk measured with triphenyltetrazolium chloride TTC, or the infarcted region using indium-111 labeled antimyosin.

This approach may be improved by new methods for the calculation of myocardial flow-extraction fraction, combined with fast T1 mapping. Taking advantage of the ultrafast acquisition of inversion-recovery and gradient recalled echo-planar sequences, a recent study by Saeed et al. presented time-course curves of myocardial signal intensity after injection of Gd-BOPTA/dimeglumine in an in vivo rat model [33]. This method clearly distinguished occlusive from reperfused regions depending on the myocardial concentration of the contrast agent and the vascular/extracellular volumes.

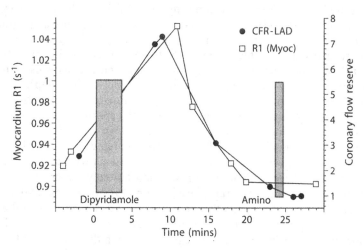

Fig. 2. Parallel variation of

$$R_1 = \frac{1}{T_1}$$

(longitudinal relaxation rate) and coronary flow velocity measured by the time-of-flight EPI technique during pharmacological stress. This type of measurement may lead to a real non invasive non radioactive assessment of coronary perfusion without injection of any contrast agent

In human studies, the role of Gd-DTPA has been evaluated by several teams in the setting of both acute and chronic ischemia. In the first week after acute MI, Holman et al. compared the extent of regions with increased signal intensity on T1 weighted images with the peak of CPK-Mb release and cumulative release of hydroxybutyrate dehydrogenase (HBDH), which are both closely related to morbidity and mortality [34]. These authors demonstrated an excellent correlation between the infarct size evaluated from the MR images and HBDH total release suggesting an accurate and possibly prognostic evaluation of the infarct extension.

Studying infarct enhancement at 1, 2, 4, and 12 weeks after AMI, Nishimura et al. showed that signal increase from gadolinium uptake is a marker of acute myocardial infarction. This enhancement, however, was no longer demonstrated in later stages suggesting that poor myocardial perfusion in scar tissue limited the distribution of Gd-GTPA. Van Dijkman also proposed an analysis of contrast enhancement with time in 84 patients diagnosed with an acute MI, and showed that improved visualization of the infarct by Gd-DTPA occurred up to 6 weeks after the acute event with a peak effect at 1 week [35].

The study of distribution patterns in acute MI discriminates regions with open arteries and regions with occluded arteries ("dark core" where contrast agent cannot diffuse due to capillary destruction). In one such study, the extension of the dark core regions correlated with both the extent of regional dysfunction and the extent of fixed thallium defects on cardiac scintigraphy. However, the simple analysis of enhancement of signal intensity may not always allow the differentiation between reperfused and non reperfused areas. De Roos illustrated this difficulty by comparing MR analysis with the patency status of the responsible artery assessed by conventional coronary angiography after thrombolytic therapy [36]. Signal intensities increased in both reperfused and non reperfused infarcted regions 15–20 min after Gd infusion (Gd-DTPA, 0.1 mM/kg body weight). The different enhancement patterns were: diffuse, subendocardial (more frequent in the nonreperfused group), hemorrhagic (with low signal intensity), or bright with a dark core. However, this study confirmed that significant signal increase of both reperfused and non reperfused areas allowed identification of acute infarction in images up to 30 min after contrast infusion. Another study by the same group demonstrated that a region of contrast enhancement was present in all patients with a myocardial infarction at 1 and 4 weeks. This region was substantially larger in nonreperfused patients as opposed to the reperfused group (15% vs 8%, $p<0.001$). Lima et al. demonstrated in 44 patients that contrast-enhanced perfusion studies predicted long-term prognosis after myocardial infarction: patients with regions of no-reflow, defined as hypoenhanced segments during the first pass of a Gadolinium bolus, had a higher rate of cardiovascular death, heart failure and reinfarction [37].

Detection of Myocardial Ischemia and Viability, Comparison with Radionuclide Techniques

Myocardial ischemia may result in three types of conditions such as stunning, hibernation (both reversible: viable myocardium) and infarction (irreversible necrosis). These states however coexist in different zones of an ischemic heart with CAD. While the third condition has no chance to evolve properly, the first two have a large potential to recover after complete revascularization (hibernation) or sufficient time (stunning). It seems that a myocardial blood flow over 0.2–0.3 ml/g/min is necessary for preserving membrane integrity and cell viability. At these flow levels, hibernating myocardium seems to match both inotropic and flow reserve at a lower level than normal.

Hartnell et al. [38] have recently shown that stress MR myocardial perfusion imaging combined with MR ventriculography provided similar accuracy to stress 99mTc-sestamibi scintigraphy in detecting myocardial ischemia of both potential and proved coronary patients. Walsh et al. using a technique derived from a "keyhole" imaging sequence (partial k-space sampling) compared perfusion indexes derived from MRI to 99mTc SPECT data in ischemic patients [39]. However, some discrepancies were found between the two methods: 28 out of 45 patients showed 100% concordance in all resting and stressed myocardial regions, but 17 did not. This appear to be related to the technical limitations specific to each technique and also to the fact that SPECT derives its signal from tissues which are both viable and perfused, whereas MRI signal intensity depends only on perfusion and capillary permeability.

There is an increasing number of puplications regarding viability testing in humans [40, 41]. Much of the information presented above could apply to the topic of viability testing, for detection of an infarction defines a region as non-viable. There have been several studies which have examined provocative testing to determine the presence of viable myocardium. Pennell et al. performed studies to evaluate coronary disease patients. In the first study 40 patients post-MI were examined, and reversible ischemia was detected using dipyridamole infusion with a sensitivity of 67% [42]. A followup study examined wall motion abnormalities using dobutamine provocation in patients with a history of myocardial infarction. A sensitivity of 91% was demonstrated for the detection of reversible ischemia. Myocardial tagging was used by Cubukcu et al. to examine patients using dobutamine challenge. They found that segment shortening agreed with thallium data, but conclusive quantitative data will require a larger patient population.

Three recent studies showed applications of MR to the assessment of myocardial contractile reserve in CAD patients. Measuring the improvement of subsegmental contractility in 15 patients by tagging, Cubukcu et al. showed that tagged cine MRI combined with low-dose dobutamine contributed to the prediction of successful revascularization [43]. In 44 patients Lima et al. demonstrated that contrast-enhanced perfusion studies predicted long-term prognosis after myocardial infarction: patients with regions with hypoenhanced segments during the first pass of a Gadolinium bolus, had a higher rate of cardiovascular death and reinfarction [37].

Future: Real-Time MRI and Dedicated Systems

A powerful MR application under development is an open magnet which permits interventional procedures to be performed under MR guidance [44]. This device is being developed for central nervous system and general body applications. Cardiac application does not appear straightforward noting that cardiac interventional procedures are frequently an extension of a diagnostic study. However, information that is not routinely available, such as chemical or physical characterization, may add to the diagnostic accuracy and predictability of outcome of a procedure. Real-time images, however, can now be acquired on conventional scanners [45], that can track an introduced catheter [46], and dedicated systems are used that add this recent progress. Finally, the combination of all the measurable informations makes the greatest potential of future MR. The combination of studies of anatomy, MR angiography, three-dimensional velocity mapping, determination of flow reserve, perfusion measurement, regional contractile reserve, metabolism and tissue characterization may provide a complete description of the cardiovascular system and its dynamics.

One of the major problem with the evaluation of cardiac NMR in its cost and benefits is that the extremely high pace of technical development quickly outdates previous conclusions. The cost for a current 1.5 T clinical system usually ranges $2 million, but lower-field systems may appear at lower cost [47]. In any case, the impact on the therapeutic decision of the determination of myocardial perfusion, function (global, regional, and segmental), metabolism and ultimately viability, and of coronary anatomy, stenoses and flow reserve, will have to be evaluated when all these technique are performed together during a single session. With this goal, faster imaging techniques and especially real-time interactive imagers, the equivalent of a non-invasive fluoroscopy, may further reduce scan times and costs and revolutionize the present feelings of physiologists and cardiologists by providing a clinical tool, that combines the easiness of ultrasound and the wealth of approaches of NMR.

References

1. Shellock FG, Kanal E, SMRI Safety Committee. Policies, guidelines, and recom mendations for MR imaging safety and patients management. J Magn Reson Imaging 1991, 1:97–101
2. Hofman MBM, Paschal CB, Debiao L et al. MRI of coronary arteries: 2D breath-hold vs. 3D respiratory-gated acquisition. J Comput Assist Tomog 1995, 19:56–62
3. Hundley WG; Hamilton CA; Clarke GD; Hillis LD; Herrington DM; Lange RA; Applegate RJ; Thomas MS; Payne J; Link KM; Peshock RM. Visualization and functional assessment of proximal and middle left anterior descending coronary stenoses in humans with magnetic resonance imaging. Circulation 1999 Jun 29;99:3248–54
4. Li D. Physical principles of magnetic resonance angiography. Coron Artery Dis 1999 May; 10:129–34
5. Keegan J; Gatehouse PD; Taylor AM; Yang GZ; Jhooti P; Firmin DN. Coronary artery imaging in a 0.5-Tesla scanner: implementation of real-time, navigator echo-controlled segmented k-space Flash and interleaved-spiral sequences. Magn Reson Med 1999;41:392–9
6. Hofman MB; Henson RE; Kovacs SJ; Fischer SE; Lauffer RB; Adzamli K; De Becker J; Wickline SA; Lorenz CH. Blood pool agent strongly improves 3D magnetic resonance coronary

angiography using an inversion pre-pulse. Magn Reson Med 1999;41:360–7

7. Slavin GS; Riederer SJ; Ehman RL. Two-dimensional multishot echo-planar coronary MR angiography. Magn Reson Med 1998;40:883–9

8. Sakuma H; Goto M; Nomura Y; Kato N; Takeda K; Higgins CB. Three-dimensional coronary magnetic resonance angiography with injection of extracellular contrast medium. Invest Radiol 1999;34:503–8

9. Double-oblique free-breathing high resolution three-dimensional coronary magnetic resonance angiography. Stuber M; Botnar RM; Danias PG; Sodickson DK Kissinger KV; Van Cauteren M; De Becker J; Manning WJ. J Am Coll Cardiol 1999 Aug;34(2):524–31

10. Cline HE; Thedens DR; Irarrazaval P; Meyer CH; Hu BS Nishimura DG; Ludke S: §D MR coronary artery segmentation. Magn Reson Med 1998;40:698–702

11. Toussaint JF, Southern JF, Fuster V, Kantor HL. T2 Contrast for NMR Characterization of Human Atherosclerosis. Arterioscl Thromb and Vasc Biol 1995, 15:1533–1542

12. Toussaint JF, LaMuraglia GM, Southern JF, Fuster V, Kantor HL. Magnetic resonance images lipid, fibrous, calcified, hemorrhagic, and thrombotic components of human atherosclerosis in vivo. Circulation 1996, 94:932–938

13. Meyer CH, Hu BS, Macovski A, Nishimura DG. Coronary vessel wall imaging. Proc Int Soc Magn Reson Med 1998, 1:15 (Abstr)

14. Fayad ZA, Fuster VF, Fallon JT, Sharma SK, Jayasundera TG, Worthley SG, Helft G, Aguinaldo G, Badimon JJ: Human coronary atherosclerotic wall imaging using in vivo high-resolution MR. Circulation, 1999; 100(18): I–520 (Abstract 2742)

15. Doorey AJ, Wills JS, Blasetto J, Goldenberg EM. Usefulness of MRI for diagnosing an anomalous coronary artery coursing between aorta and pulmonary trunk. Am J Cardiol 1994, 74:198–199

16. McConnell MV, Ganz P, Selwyn AP, Edelman RR, Manning WJ. Identification of anomalous coronary arteries and their anatomic course by Magnetic Resonance coronary angiography. Circulation 1995, 92:3158–3162

17. Post JC, van Rossum AC, Bronzwaer JGF et al. Magnetic resonance angiography of anomalous coronary arteries. A new gold standard for delineating the proximal course? Circulation 1995, 92:3163–3171

18. Edelman RR, Manning WJ, Gervino E, and Li W. Flow velocity quantification in human coronary arteries with fast, breath-hold angiography. J Magn Reson Imaging 1993, 3:699–703

19. Poncelet BP, Weisskoff RM, Wedeen VJ, Brady TJ, Kantor H. Time of flight quantification of coronary flow with echo-planar MRI. Magn Reson Med 1993, 30:447–457

20. Gonzalez F, Bassingthwaighte JB. Heterogeneities in regional volumes of distribution and flows in rabbit heart. Am J Physiol 1990, 258:H1012-H1024

21. Wilke N, Simm C, Zhang J et al. Contrast enhanced first pass myocardial perfusion imaging: Correlation between myocardial blood flow in dogs at rest and during hyperemia. Magn Reson Med 1993, 29:485–497

22. Kivelitz DE, Bis KG, Wilke NM. Quantitative MR first-pass vs. N13-ammonia PET in coronary artery disease. Radiology 1997, 205:253–254

23. Fritz-Hansen T; Rostrup E; Sondergaard L; Ring PB; Amtorp O; Larsson HB. Capillary transfer constant of Gd-DTPA in the myocardium at rest and during vasodilation assessed by MRI. Magn Reson Med 1998;40:922–9

24. Lima JAC, Judd RM, Olivieri CL, Schulman SP, Atalar E, Zerhouni EA. Myocardial perfusion by contrast enhanced ultrafast MRI relates to myocardial damage in patients with acute myocardial infarction. Proc Soc Magn Reson 1994, 1:109

25. Niemi P, Poncelet BP, Kwong KK; Weisskoff RM; Rosen BR; Brady TJ; Kantor HL: Myocardial intensity changes associated with flow stimulation in blood oxygenation sensitive magnetic resonance imaging. Magn Reson Med 1996;36:78–82

26. Li D, Dhawale P, Haacke EM, Rubin PJ, Gropler RJ. Myocardial BOLD effects of dipyridamole and dobutamine using a segmented double-echo interleaved sequence. Proc Soc Magn Reson 1995, 1:339

27. Detre JA, Leigh JS, Williams DS, Koretsky AP. Perfusion Imaging. Magn Reson Med 1992, 23:37–45

28. Walsh EG, Minematsu K, Leppo J, Moore SC. Radioactive microsphere validation of a volume localized continuous saturation perfusion measurement. Magn Reson Med 1994, 31:147–153

29. Balaban RS, Taylor JF, Turner R. Effect of cardiac flow on gradient recalled echo images of the canine heart. NMR Biomed 1994, 7:89–95

30. Judd RM, Atalay MK, Rottman GA, Zerhouni EA. Effects of myocardial water exchange on T1 enhancement during bolus administration of MR contrast agents. Magn Reson Med 1995, 33:215–223

31. Toussaint JF, Kwong KK, M'Kparu F et al. Perfusion Changes in Human Skeletal Muscle During Reactive Hyperemia Measured by Echo-Planar Imaging. Magn Reson Med 1996, 35:62–69

32. Ovize M, Pichard JB, de Lorgeril M, et al. Accurate quantitation of infarct size by Gd-DOTA enhanced magnetic resonance imaging in the dog. J Am Coll Cardiol 1991, 17:242 A

33. Saeed M, Wendland MF, Yu KK, et al. Identification of myocardial reperfusion with echo planar MRI. Circulation 1994, 90:1492–1501

34. Holman ER, van Jonbergen HPW, van Dijkman PRM, van der Laarse A, de Roos A, van der Wall EE. Comparison of MRI studies with enzymatic indexes of myocardial necrosis for quantification of myocardial infarct size. Am J Cardiol 1993, 71:1036–1040

35. Van Dijkman PRM, Van der Wall EE, De Roos A, et al. Acute, subacute, and chronic myocardial infarction: quantitative analysis of Gadolinium-enhanced MR images. Radiology 1991, 180:147–151

36. De Roos A, Van Rossum AC, Van der Wall EE, et al. Reperfused and nonreperfused myocardial infarction: potential of Gd-DTPA enhanced MRI. Radiology 1989, 172:717–720

37. Lima JAC, Wu K, Judd RM et al. Infarct extent and presence of no-reflow regions by contrast enhanced MRI predict long-term prognosis after acute myocardial infarction. Circulation 1995, 92:I-509

38. Hartnell G, Cerel A, Kamalesh M et al. Detection of myocardial ischemia: Value of combined myocardial perfusion and cineangiographic MR imaging. Am J Roentgenol 1994, 163:1061–1067

39. Walsh EG, Doyle M, Lawson MA, Blackwell GG, Pohost GM. Multislice first-pass myocardial perfusion imaging on a conventional clinical scanner. Magn Reson Med 1995, 34:39–47

40. Dendale P; Franken PR; Holman E; Avenarius J; van der Wall EE; de Roos A. Validation of low-dose dobutamine magnetic resonance imaging for assessment of myocardial viability after infarction by serial imaging. Am J Cardiol 1998;82:375–7

41. Baer FM; Theissen P; Schneider CA; Voth E; Sechtem U; Schicha H; Erdmann E. Dobutamine magnetic resonance imaging predicts contractile recovery of chronically dysfunctional myocardium after sucessful revascularization. J Am Coll Cardiol 1998;31:1040–8

42. Pennell DJ. Underwood SR. Ell PJ. Swanton RH. Walker JM. Longmore DB. Dipyridamole magnetic resonance imaging: a comparison with thallium-201 emission tomography. Br Heart J. 1990, 64:362–369

43. Cubukcu AA, Ridgway JP, Sivananthan UM et al. Detection of contractile reserve by tagged cine MRI during low-dose dobutamine infusion. Circulation 1995, 92:I-508

44. Schenck J, Jolesz F, Roemer P, Cline HE, Lorensen WE, Kikinis R et al. Superconducting open-configuration MR imaging system for image-guided therapy. Radiology 1995, 195:805–814

45. Kerr AB, Pauly JM, Hu B et al. Real-time Interactive MRI on a conventional scanner. Magn Reson Med 1997, 38:355–367

46. Unal O, Korosec F, Frayne R, Strother C, Mistretta C. A rapid 2D time-resolved variable-rate k-space sampling MR technique for passive catheter tracking during endovascular procedures. Magn Reson Med 1998, 40:356–362

47. Macovski A, Conolly S. Novel approaches to low-cost MRI. Magn Reson Med 1993, 30:221–230

Section IV:
Therapeutic and Clinical Applications

Intracoronary Ultrasound Imaging

J.-C. Tardif and J. Grégoire

Introduction

Intracoronary ultrasound (ICUS) imaging uses miniaturized transducers at the tip of catheters to supply tomographic, cross-sectional images of coronary arteries [1, 2]. ICUS provides detailed information not only on the degree of arterial stenosis but also on the atherosclerotic lesions and the vessel wall [3]. The traditional angiographic approach used to evaluate coronary artery disease has well-known limitations. One shortcoming is that coronary angiography provides only a planar perspective of the arterial lumen. Depiction of the coronary lumen, and not the wall, is another important limitation of angiography, atherosclerosis being primarily a disease of the arterial wall. The severity of stenosis may be underestimated by angiography because the reference segment used to quantitate the lesion is involved in the diffuse atherosclerotic process. In addition, the composition and morphology of atherosclerotic lesions, which cannot be assessed with angiography, are major determinants of the clinical expression of coronary atherosclerosis and of the response to percutaneous interventions.

Intracoronary Ultrasound Instrumentation

Because high-frequency ultrasound transducers have greater resolution, 20–50 MHz transducers on 2.6–3.5 French catheters are employed for ICUS imaging. These catheters use either mechanical or solid-state (multi-element) designs. Several types of mechanical instruments exist, but they basically consist in a drive shaft which is connected to a motor that rotates a single, small ultrasound element. In contrast, solid-state catheters use up to 64 elements activated in sequence. Dynamic focusing is achieved electronically in a solid-state system to create a synthetic aperture that results in optimal focus in both the near and far fields. Since a drive shaft is not required with multi-element systems, it is possible to use the central lumen of the catheter for other purposes. In addition, the absence of rotating components in a solid-state system prevents potential artefacts due to nonuniform rotational distortion (NURD) that may occur with mechanical systems. On the other hand, the acoustic power of older multi-element systems was limited and the central ringdown artifact used to be large. However, both types of designs have been improved by manufacturers in the recent years and they are now relatively equivalent for all clinical and research purposes [4]. Instruments that combine ultrasound with other capabilities such as a balloon angioplasty catheter or an atherectomy device have been developed to facilitate guidance of interventions [5, 6]. Interestingly, an imaging guidewire has recently been produced by one manufacturer [7]. A limitation common to all these intracoronary instruments is the lack of forward-viewing capability. A prototype catheter that allows visualization beyond the catheter tip has recently been developed [8].

Intracoronary Ultrasound Examination

The procedure is performed by advancing the ICUS catheter distal to the site of interest to an easily recognizable landmark, most often a side branch, using a 0.014 or 0.018 inch coronary angioplasty guidewire. Intracoronary nitroglycerin is administered (150–300 μg) before the examination. The most distal position of the ICUS catheter is noted and used for follow-up examinations. It is recommended that the guiding catheter be disengaged to ensure visualization of the aorto-ostial junction by ultrasound imaging. The transducer is then pullbacked automatically at a speed of 0.5 (or 1.0) mm/s, up to the guiding catheter. The use of reproducible landmarks and a known pullback speed facilitates comparison of identical cross-sectional images on serial studies and permits volumetric (three-dimensional) analysis. Alternatively, slow manual pullbacks (approximately 0.5 mm/s) can be performed up to the guiding catheter. A detailed running audio commentary describing the location of the ongoing ICUS interrogation and of areas of interest is extremely useful with either type of pullback. Simultaneous high-resolution fluoroscopic images can also be recorded on the ICUS imaging screen during pullbacks to constantly know the location of the ultrasound transducer. ICUS images are usually recorded only during transducer pullback and not during transducer advancement to ease off-line image interpretation.

For safe imaging of coronary arteries, the ICUS catheter must be small and flexible enough to allow passage in tortuous vessels. Although miniaturization of catheters has taken place in the past years (2.6–3.5 French, 0.7–1.1 mm), it occasionally remains not possible to cross severe narrowings before angioplasty. Major complications are rare despite increasing clinical use of ICUS imaging [9]. Most major and acute procedural complications associated with (but not necessarily caused by) ICUS imaging occur during interventional cases. Coronary spasm occurs in approximately 2–3% of patients during interventional and diagnostic catheterization but it usually can be reversed rapidly by the administration of nitroglycerin. Importantly, heparin (5000–10,000 U) should be administered before ICUS examination even for diagnostic imaging. The 1-year safety of intracoronary ultrasound imaging has been assessed by serial quantitative coronary angiography in 38 cardiac transplant recipients [10]. There was no significant difference between instrumented and noninstrumented vessels in percentage or absolute change in diameter 1 year after the initial ICUS examination.

Assessment of Vascular Anatomy
and Pathology with ICUS

ICUS measurements of vascular dimensions have been shown by several investigators to correlate closely with histologic measurements [11]. When an internal layer is visualized with ICUS, its normal thickness does not exceed 0.20 mm. An intermediate echolucent zone is observed in 60–70% of patients. When this middle layer is present, its thickness is also 0.20 mm or less. A third layer, outside the external elastic membrane (junction of media and adventitia), is present but its thickness can rarely be defined in native vessels because of surrounding tissues. Abnormalities of the arterial lumen and wall are depicted in details by ICUS [12] (Fig. 1). Histologically, progressive accumulation of plaque in the intima is often associated with disruption of the internal elastic lamina and increased collagen content in the media. The resulting modifications in the echogenicity of these structures may render difficult the identification of the intimal-medial border [13]. The interface between lumen and intima and the border between media and adventitia (the external elastic membrane) however remain easily discernable and reliable. For these reasons, quantitative analysis on ICUS cross-sections consists in measurements of lumen area and of the area circumscribed by the external elastic membrane (Fig. 2). The difference between these two areas is the intima + plaque area, i.e. the wall area apart from the surrounding adventitia.

ICUS imaging provides characterization of the vessel wall based on tissue reflectivity and not on histology per se. Depending of the composition of the atheroma and of the changes in the vascular wall, different patterns will be observed on the ICUS image. Calcium causes the greatest impedance to transmission of ultrasound, resulting in considerable reflection with minimal penetration

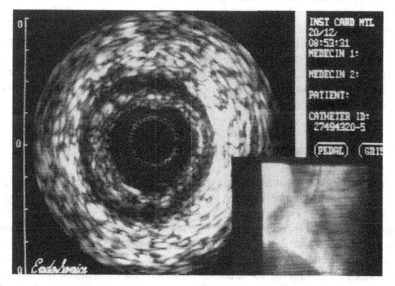

Fig. 1. Mild to moderate atherosclerotic plaque seen with ICUS

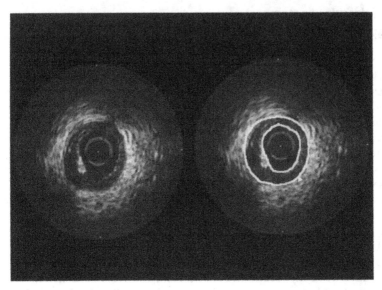

Fig. 2. Illustration of ICUS measurements. The inner and outer white lines indicate lumen and external elastic membrane areas, respectively

of ultrasound signals. Calcium deposits in atherosclerotic plaques are very bright and cause acoustic shadowing. Fibrous plaques are bright but do not cause acoustic shadowing. Atheroma rich in lipids ("soft plaque") and lesions composed of proliferating smooth muscle cells and extracellular matrix are less echogenic than the surrounding adventitia and less than fibrous or calcified plaque. An heterogeneous appearance is frequently present in atheromatous arteries, because they often contain a combination of lipid-laden, fibrous and calcified plaques. ICUS also allows the identification of necrotic debris and lipid lakes. Arterial thrombus can be detected with ICUS, but distinction between soft plaque and thrombus can be difficult. Interestingly, one study has shown that this classification of plaque morphology by ICUS correlated very well with the clinical angina syndrome, but not with the angiographic lesion descriptors [14]. In that study, patients with unstable angina had more soft plaques and less fibrous and calcified plaques.

ICUS Versus Coronary Angiography

The limitations of coronary arteriography are now well known [2, 15]. The planar, two-dimensional silhouette of the arterial lumen provided by coronary angiography and the lack of depiction of the arterial wall are the most important limitations. Because the lesion is assessed by comparing the lumen of the narrowed and "normal" segments, disease of the reference segment and compensatory enlargement (arterial remodeling or Glagov phenomenon [16]) of the stenosed segment frequently lead to angiographic underestimation of the extent and severity of coronary artery disease. The study of mildly diseased coronary arteries has revealed that half of the patients with such angiographic results have narrowings of 50% or more with ICUS [17]. Moreover, the majority of angiographically normal reference segments are involved in the atherosclerotic process on ICUS imaging [18].

Visual interpretation of arteriograms is associated with significant intra-observer and inter-observer variability. The advent of quantitative coronary angiography has reduced this variability, but it has not improved the ability of the radiographic two-dimensional silhouette of the arterial lumen to accurately depict complex tridimensional coronary anatomy. Correlations between ICUS and angiographic measurements vary depending on the presence or absence of atherosclerotic disease, the eccentricity of lesions, the performance of an interventional procedure, and the index measured [2, 19, 20]. In normal subjects, the correlations between angiographic and ultrasound diameters are excellent. However, the correlations are not as good in patients with atheromatous vessels. The presence of tortuous arteries, vessel overlap, stenoses at bifurcations and eccentric lesion morphology compound the problem of reliable depiction of the coronary lumen.

An imperfect correlation is noted between ICUS and angiography in the evaluation of residual stenosis and luminal areas after angioplasty [21]. These differences are probably due to the larger angiographic diameters caused by the presence of contrast in fissures in the arterial wall, whereas the tomographic sections on ICUS precisely depict the true architecture and dimensions of the arterial lumen. Serious underestimation of residual plaque burden at the dilated site after a percutaneous intervention frequently occurs when only angiographic monitoring is used, with cross-sectional area narrowings of 60% or significantly more being commonly present on ICUS [22] (Fig. 3).

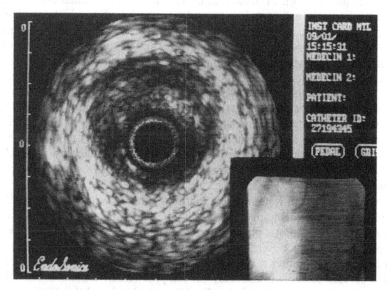

Fig. 3. Severe residual plaque burden on ICUS, despite "good" angiographic results of balloon angioplasty

Diagnostic Applications of Intracoronary Ultrasound

Clinical indications for ICUS are evolving. One important application of ICUS during diagnostic catheterization is for the evaluation of left main coronary artery disease, when doubts persist after angiography [23]. This particularly occurs when a diagnostic catheter repetitively wedges in the left coronary artery, when the left main trunk is diffusely small without any discrete lesion or when an ostial lesion or a stenosis at the bifurcation is suspected. In order to assess the left main coronary artery adequately, the ICUS catheter is first advanced in the left anterior descending or circumflex artery, the guiding catheter is disengaged and ultrasound imaging is performed up to the guiding catheter to ensure visualization of the aorto-ostial junction. If a significant lesion is not observed in the left main artery in this fashion, we frequently instrument the other major coronary branch (i.e. the circumflex artery if the guidewire was initially introduced in the left anterior descending artery) and image its proximal portion to rule out the presence of a left main equivalent disease (severe ostial narrowings of circumflex and LAD). Although ICUS provides anatomic depiction of narrowings and not a physiologic assessment, it nevertheless clarifies the vast majority of problematic angiographic images of the left main artery. Indeed, ICUS imaging in this context will often show minimal plaque accumulation or very severe narrowing. In intermediate cases with at least moderate disease, we rely on several off-line ultrasound measurements performed immediately after imaging is completed. We first require the presence of a cross-sectional area narrowing greater than 75% before considering that a lesion is "significant". We also measure the true minimal lumen diameter (MLD) and divide it by the lumen diameter of a normal left main segment if present, to obtain a percent diameter stenosis. This is particularly useful in ostial lesions and in heavily calcified arteries (causing shadowing of the external elastic membrane area). In diffusely diseased left main coronary arteries, we also divide the MLD by the expected normal dimension of the left main artery (based on autopsy series and angiographic studies of normal patients). A greater than 50% diameter stenosis is taken to represent a significant stenosis. It is important to stress that these values have not been specifically validated for use in this context. Nevertheless, experimental obstruction to coronary flow in animals has shown that coronary flow reserve begins to be significantly limited with a cross-sectional area narrowing of 75% [24], which roughly corresponds to a 50% diameter stenosis. We have also recently demonstrated that a cross-sectional area narrowing of 75% or more in a coronary artery on ICUS correlates very well with the presence of ST segment depression during treadmill testing [25].

Other ambiguous lesions on angiography can also be clarified with ICUS [26]. Indeed, the value of angiography is more limited at coronary bifurcations. Unfortunately, atherosclerotic plaques preferentially accumulate at bifurcation points, where turbulence is more important. Bifurcation lesions of uncertain severity thus represent another diagnostic application of ICUS. Ultrasound imaging can also provide valuable information for the problematic lesions visualized well in only a single angiographic projection. We have also found that ICUS is helpful in patients with chest pain in the first 6 months after angioplasty to determine whether a severe narrowing is present despite the absence of significant angiographic restenosis [25]. Because ICUS does not provide functional assessment of lesions, the narrowings of truly intermediate severity however can benefit from Doppler assessment of the flow reserve [27].

Coronary vasculopathy is the leading cause of late mortality following cardiac transplantation. A high prevalence of false negative coronary arteriograms has been documented with the use of ICUS during routine serial catheterization in cardiac transplant recipients [28]. Concentric intimal thickening is often not detected by angiography because of the diffuse nature of this immune process. In contrast, ICUS imaging offers early detection and quantitation of coronary vasculopathy in patients who have undergone cardiac transplantation [29]. The presence of significant intimal thickening on ICUS has been shown to be predictive of survival in these patients, even in the absence of angiographically apparent disease [30]. The use of ICUS may therefore allow the early use of more effective treatment strategies in cardiac transplant recipients. Interestingly, ICUS imaging performed within a few weeks of transplantation has revealed the presence of angiographically silent focal atherosclerotic plaques in 25–30% of patients [31]. These plaques most likely represent disease transferred from the donor.

ICUS can also allow for the characterization of other coronary syndromes (syndrome X, myocardial bridging, coronary artery spasm). The majority of patients with syndrome X have abnormal coronary arteries (atheroma or marked intimal thickening) by ICUS imaging, despite the absence of angiographic abnormalities [32]. Similarly, a very high incidence of atherosclerotic plaque is detected proximal to bridging segments with the use of ICUS [33]. Occasionally, these plaques are sufficiently important to justify angioplasty. Controversy however persists concerning the clinical significance of myocardial bridging. Finally, marked atherosclerotic thickening is generally demonstrated by ICUS at the site of focal coronary vasospasm in the absence of angiographically significant disease [34].

Applications of ICUS During Coronary Interventions

ICUS has been extremely useful to understand the mechanisms of lumen enlargement with different percutaneous coronary interventions. We have learned that the improvement in lumen dimensions after balloon angioplasty was predominantly the result of both vascular expansion (increase in the area circumscribed by the external elastic membrane, particularly for compliant non-calcified plaques), and dissection [35]. We have also realized that plaque could be redistributed along the long-axis of the vessel. On the other hand, ICUS has shown that extraction of plaque is the principal mechanism for lumen enlargement after atherectomy [36].

ICUS is a more sensitive tool than fluoroscopy to detect coronary calcifications in patients in whom angioplasty is required (75% vs 48% in one study) [37]. The extent (number of quadrants, axial length) and localization (superficial or deep) of these calcifications can be precisely defined with ICUS. Calcification of the culprit coronary lesion is a determinant of the response to interventions [38]. Directional atherectomy does not remove calcium very well and the presence of more than mild calcification represents a contraindication to its use. In contrast, rotational atherectomy results in preferential ablation of calcified lesions. Balloon angioplasty may cause dissection at calcified lesions, particularly at the junction with a more normal wall. ICUS can also depict plaque eccentricity at the stenosis site more reliably than angiography [39]. Although the GUIDE trial investigators have reported that such ICUS findings (calcifications, plaque eccentricity) have resulted in changes in therapy in approximately 50% of their patients [40], reductions in restenosis rates have unfortunately not been reported.

Sizing of instruments is usually based on the lumen dimensions of the reference segments. The indiscriminate use of balloons larger than the angiographic reference segment lumen has resulted in a high rate of complications after balloon angioplasty. However, it has been demonstrated that angiography significantly underestimates plaque burden of the reference segment because of adaptive vascular remodeling, the process whereby compensatory vessel enlargement develops to preserve the arterial lumen. There is, on average, approximately 50% cross-sectional area narrowing on ICUS at angiographic "reference" segments [18]. The CLOUT Pilot Trial investigators have shown that remodeled arteries (as shown by ICUS) can safely accomodate oversized balloons [41]. In that study, balloons sized halfway between the lumen and external elastic membrane resulted in upsizing in 73% of cases, by an average of 0.5 mm compared to angioplasty guided by angiography. This increased the nominal balloon-to-artery ratio from 1.12 to 1.30 and the minimal lumen diameter on ICUS from 1.75 to 2.10 mm. Interestingly, these results were obtained without increased rates of complications. Whether this strategy will result in lower restenosis rates and improved long-term outcomes is not known. However, phase 2 of the GUIDE Trial has shown that a residual percent plaque area of less than 65% and a minimal lumen diameter of more than 2.0 mm on ICUS were associated with a low likelihood of restenosis [42]. Given the strong predictive value of post-procedural plaque area on ICUS, it is tempting to speculate that ultrasound guidance during interventions to reduce residual atheroma will translate into better long-term outcome. Data supporting this hypothesis is now emerging. Careful ICUS guidance of directional atherectomy and adjunct PTCA in the ABACAS trial resulted in a residual plaque area of 42%, and a restenosis rate of 14% (at 3 months) [43]. In comparison, final plaque burden was 58% in the Optimal Atherectomy Restenosis Study, and the restenosis rate was 29% [44]. Thus, lowering residual plaque burden by using ultrasound guidance may have been responsible for the decrease in restenosis rate in the ABACAS trial.

True lumen dimensions at the dilated site are defined more accurately with the tomographic images obtained with ICUS than with angiography, particularly when there is nonhomogeneous contrast density or when vessel borders are indistinct. The causes of angiographic haziness can usually be identified with ICUS. Surface ulcerations and dissections are detected more frequently with ICUS than with angiography. However, there are presently no criteria to distinguish the dissections that are useful from those which are detrimental with ICUS.

ICUS has dramatically changed the world of coronary artery stenting. Colombo et al. initially demonstrated that stent deployment was commonly sub-optimal on ICUS despite an apparently adequate expansion on angiography [45]. It was then shown that oral anticoagulation was not necessary to prevent subacute thrombosis when deployment was optimized using strict ICUS criteria [46]. Optimization of stent deployment according to ICUS criteria usually involved the agressive use of high-pressure balloon inflations. Building on the knowledge acquired with ICUS, other investigators then obtained favorable results with systematic high-pressure inflations, without using ICUS or coumadin [47, 48]. This led to a controversy regarding the need for and cost-effectiveness of the continued use of ICUS during stenting. However, angiographic criteria predicting adequate stent expansion on ICUS have not been developed [49]. In addition, some investigators argue that ICUS has demonstrated that inflations at very high pressures are not always necessary to obtain adequate stent deployment and sometimes may only lead to injury at stent edges. Such injuries in turn will often require the use of additional balloon inflations or the deployment of one or more additional stents. Randomized, multicenter clinical trials have been initiated to reassess the role of ICUS in coronary stenting (AVID, OPTICUS).

Full apposition of the stent to the arterial wall represents one of the most important ICUS criterion of adequate deployment (Fig. 4). Experienced observers also visually assess the relationship between the proximal and distal portions of the stent and their adjacent reference segments. Quantitative criteria usually involve a symetry index (ratio of minimal to maximal lumen diameters on the same cross-section greater than 0.7) and ratios of the minimal intra-stent luminal area and lumen areas of the reference segments. For example, the criteria used in the MUSIC trial were rigid and required that the smallest lumen area in the stent was both 100% or more of the lumen area of the smallest reference segment (90% if minimal intra-stent luminal area ≥ 9 mm^2) and 90% of the average of the lumen areas of the

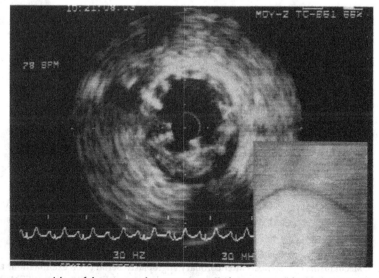

Fig. 4. Inadequate apposition of the stent to the coronary wall (from 6 to 8 o'clock) demonstrated by ICUS

references (80% if minimal intra-stent luminal area ≥ 9 mm^2) [50]. Most investigators presently use quantitative criteria that are slightly less stringent.

Several pharmacologic approaches have failed to modify the high incidence of restenosis after balloon coronary angioplasty. This inability to alter the restenosis process was in part caused by our incomplete understanding of its pathophysiology. It was assumed for several years that restenosis was solely caused by intimal hyperplasia. ICUS has allowed for a better understanding of the mechanisms responsible for restenosis after angioplasty in humans (Fig. 5). Our and other groups of investigators have shown using serial ICUS examinations that lumen loss after balloon angioplasty is caused by the combination of inadequate or deleterious vessel remodeling and neointimal formation [51–53]. Vascular remodeling is defined in this context as the change in external elastic membrane area. Importantly, ICUS has also taught us that an important residual plaque burden after angioplasty is an important contributor to restenosis in patients. In contrast, Hoffmann et al. have shown that the difficult problem of in-stent restenosis is caused by tissue hyperplasia [54] and that there is no significant chronic stent recoil at follow-up ICUS examination.

The emerging role of vascular remodeling in the pathophysiology of restenosis after coronary interventions not involving stents has created a new target for its prevention [55]. Indeed, we recently demonstrated that the antioxidant probucol prevents restenosis after coronary angioplasty by improving vascular remodeling [52, 56]. The exciting concept of a "vessel remodeler" has thus largely arisen because of the use of ICUS imaging. In comparison, radiation therapy does not appear to improve adaptive vessel enlargement but rather seems to be effective at inhibiting neointimal formation [57, 58].

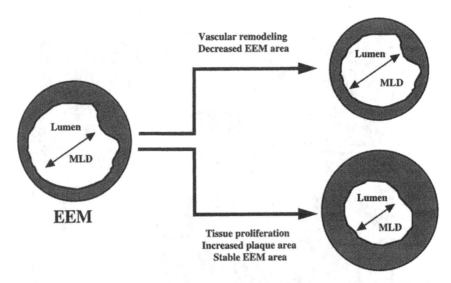

Fig. 5. Mechanisms of restenosis after coronary angioplasty. Serial ICUS examinations allow for the assessment of neointima formation and vascular remodeling in patients. EEM=External elastic membrane; MLD=Minimal lumen diameter

Research Applications of Intracoronary Ultrasound

The precise assessment of the extent of plaque burden by ICUS makes it the ideal tool for clinical trials of regression of atherosclerosis [59]. Clinical studies with lipid-lowering agents have resulted in small angiographic improvement but drastic reductions in clinical events [60]. This apparent paradox may be due, in addition to improvement of endothelial function, to the poor sensitivity of arteriography to detect changes in plaque burden in the presence of bidirectional remodeling. Quantitative analysis of two-dimensional ICUS images in future regression trials will require the selection of several cross-sections which needs to be carefully matched at baseline and at follow-up. Three-dimensional reconstruction of ICUS images using dedicated systems and software will also be used to derive the changes in plaque volume over time in coronary segments measuring 20–40 mm [61]. Three-dimensional analysis is also being used for the assessment of in-stent restenosis [54] and of its prevention. Technical requirements and present limitations of three-dimensional ICUS are beyond the scope of this chapter [62].

The elastic properties of the coronary arterial wall can also be assessed with ICUS. This method called elastography uses computer processing of the radiofrequency signals. Finally, although this chapter has dealt with spatial information provided by ICUS, temporal correlation of ultrasound images can provide information on blood velocity and on actual volume flow.

In summary, intracoronary ultrasound has the ability to complement angiography by providing cross-sectional views of the arterial lumen and by allowing for a direct in vivo assessment of the arterial wall. Its present diagnostic indications include the evaluation of ambiguous lesions, particularly in the left main coronary artery and at bifurcations. Clinical applications of ultrasound guidance during percutaneous coronary interventions primarily aim at reducing the residual plaque burden at the dilated site and at confirming adequate stent deployment. Intracoronary ultrasound has also allowed researchers to gain important insights into the mechanisms leading to restenosis after angioplasty and the antirestenotic effects of antioxidants and brachytherapy. Intracoronary ultrasound will also become the gold standard in clinical trials assessing the prevention of progression of atherosclerosis. Finally, important research efforts will be devoted to characterization of plaques using intracoronary ultrasound in the coming years.

References

1. Tardif JC, Pandian NG (1995) Intravascular and intracardiac ultrasound. Coronary Artery Disease 6:35–42
2. Tardif JC, Pandian NG (1994) Intravascular ultrasound imaging in peripheral arterial and coronary artery disease. Current Opinion in Cardiology 9:627–633
3. Pandian NG, Kreis A, Weintraub A, et al. (1990) Real-time intravascular ultrasound imaging in humans. Am J Cardiol 65:1392–1396
4. Tardif JC, Bilodeau L, Doucet S, Bonan R, Côté G (1995) Comparison between mechanical and phased-array designs for intravascular ulrasound in stented and non-stented coronary arteries: Animal studies. Circulation 92:I-600 (Abst)
5. Mudra H, Klauss V, Blasini R, et al. (1994) Ultrasound guidance of Palmaz-Schatz intracoronary stenting with a combined intravascular ultrasound balloon catheter. Circulation 90:1252–1261

6. Fitzgerald PJ, Belef M, Connolly AJ, Sudhir K, Yock PG (1995) Design and initial testing of an ultrasound-guided directional atherectomy device. Am Heart J 129:593–598
7. Moussa I, Di Mario C, Moses J, et al. (1997) Coronary stenting after rotational atherectomy in calcified and complex lesions. Circulation 96:128–136
8. Evans JL, Ng Kok-Hwee, Vonesh MJ, et al. (1994) Arterial imaging with a new forward-viewing intravascular ultrasound catheter. Circulation 89:712–717
9. Hausmann D, Erbel R, Alibelli-Chemarin MJ, et al. (1995) The safety of intracoronary ultrasound. A multicenter survey of 2207 examinations. Circulation 91:623–630
10. Pinto FJ, St Goar FG, Gao SZ, et al. (1993) Immediate and one-year safety of intracoronary ultrasonic imaging. Evaluation with serial quantitative angiography. Circulation 88:1709–1714
11. Liebson PR, Klein LW (1992) Intravascular ultrasound in coronary atherosclerosis: A new approach to clinical assessment. Am Heart J 123:1643–1660
12. Waller BF, Pinkerton CA, Slack JD (1992) Intravascular ultrasound: A histological study of vessels during life. Circulation 85:2305–2310
13. Porter TR, Radio SJ, Anderson JA, Michels A, Xie F (1994) Composition of coronary atherosclerotic plaque in the intima and media affects intravascular ultrasound measurements of intimal thickness. J Am Coll Cardiol 23:1079–1084
14. Hodgson J, Reddy KG, Suneja R, Nair RN, Lesnefsky EJ, Sheehan HM (1993) Intracoronary ultrasound imaging: correlation of plaque morphology with angiography, clinical syndrome and procedural results in patients undergoing coronary angioplasty. J Am Coll Cardiol 21:35–44
15. Vlodaver Z, Frech R, van Tassel RA, Edwards JE (1973) Correlation of the antemortem coronary angiogram and the postmortem specimen. Circulation 47:162–169
16. Glagov S, Weisenberg E, Zarins CK, et al. (1987) Compensatory enlargement of human atherosclerotic coronary arteries. N Engl J Med 316:1371–1375
17. Porter TR, Sears T, Xie F, et al. (1993) Intravascular ultrasound study of angiographically mildly diseased coronary arteries. J Am Coll Cardiol 22:1858–1865.
18. Mintz GS, Painter JA, Pichard AD, et al. (1995) Atherosclerosis in angiographically "normal" coronary artery reference segments: An intravascular ultrasound study with clinical correlations. J Am Coll Cardiol 25:1479–1485
19. De Scheerder I, De Man F, Herregods MC, et al. (1994) Intravascular ultrasound versus angiography for measurement of luminal diameters in normal and diseased coronary arteries. Am Heart J 127:243–251
20. Nissen SE, Gurley JC, Grines CL, et al. (1991) Intravascular ultrasound assessment of lumen size and wall morphology in normal subjects and coronary artery disease patients. Circulation 84:1087–1099
21. Nakamura S, Mahon DJ, Maheswaran B, et al. (1995) An explanation for discrepancy between angiographic and intravascular ultrasound measurements after percutaneous transluminal coronary angioplasty. J Am Coll Cardiol 25:633–639
22. Tobis JM, Mallery J, Mahon D, et al. (1991) Intravascular ultrasound imaging of human coronary arteries in vivo. Circulation 83:913–926
23. Pande AK, Tardif JC, Doucet S, et al. (1996) Intravascular ultrasound diagnosis of left main coronary artery stenosis. Can J Cardiol 12:757–759
24. Wilson RF (1996) Assessing the severity of coronary-artery stenoses. N Engl J Med 334:1735–1737
25. Rodes J, Malekianpour M, Tardif JC, et al. (1997) Exercise electrocardiography for the detection of restenosis after coronary angioplasty: Insights from intravascular ultrasound. Circulation 96:I-462 (Abst)
26. White CJ, Ramee SR, Collins TJ, et al. (1992) Ambiguous coronary angiography: clinical utility of intravascular ultrasound. Cathet Cardiovasc Diagn 26:200–203
27. Miller DD, Donohue TJ, Younis LT, et al. (1994) Correlation of pharmacologic 99m-Tc-sestamibi myocardial perfusion imaging with poststenotic coronary flow reserve in patients with angiographically intermediate coronary artery stenoses. Circulation 89:2150–2160

28. St Goar FG, Pinto FJ, Alderman EL, et al. (1992) Intracoronary ultrasound in cardiac transplant recipients. In vivo evidence of "angiographically silent" intimal thickening. Circulation 85:979–987
29. Pinto FJ, Chenzbraun A, Botas J, et al. (1994) Feasibility of serial intracoronary ultrasound imaging for assessment of progression of intimal proliferation in cardiac transplant recipients. Circulation 90:2348–2355
30. Rickenbacker PR, Pinto FJ, Lewis NP, et al. (1995) Prognostic importance of intimal thickness as measured by intracoronary ultrasound after cardiac transplantation. Circulation 92:3445–3452
31. Tuczu EM, Hobbs RE, Rincon G, et al. (1995) Occult and frequent transmission of atherosclerotic coronary disease with cardiac transplantation: insights from intravascular ultrasound. Circulation 91:1706–1713
32. Wiedermann JG, Schwartz A, Apfelbaum M (1995) Anatomic and physiologic heterogeneity in patients with syndrome X: An intravascular ultrasound study. J Am Coll Cardiol 25:1310–1317
33. Ge J, Erbel R, Rupprecht HJ, et al. (1994) Comparison of intravascular ultrasound and angiography in the assessment of myocardial bridging. Circulation 89:1725–1732.
34. Yamagishi M, Miyatake K, Tamai J, et al. (1994) Intravascular ultrasound detection of atherosclerosis at the site of focal vasospasm in angiographically normal or minimally narrowed coronary segments. J Am Coll Cardiol 23:352–357
35. Tenaglia AN, Buller CE, Kisslo KB, et al. (1992) Mechanisms of balloon angioplasty and directional coronary atherectomy as assessed by intracoronary ultrasound. J Am Coll Cardiol 20:685–691
36. Braden GA, Herrington DM, Downes TR, et al. (1994) Qualitative and quantitative contrasts in the mechanisms of lumen enlargement by coronary balloon angioplasty and directional coronary atherectomy. J Am Coll Cardiol 23:40–48
37. Mintz GS, Douek P, Pichard AD, et al. (1992) Target lesion calcification in coronary artery disease: an intravascular ultrasound study. J Am Coll Cardiol 20:1149–1155
38. Mintz GS, Pichard AD, Kovach JA, et al. (1994) Impact of preintervention intravascular ultrasound imaging on transcatheter treatment strategies in coronary artery disease. Am J Cardiol 73:423–430
39. Mintz GS, Popma JJ, Pichard AD, et al. (1996) Limitations of angiography in the assessment of plaque distribution in coronary disease. Circulation 93:924–931
40. GUIDE trial Investigators (1993) Impact of intravascular ultrasound on device selection and endpoint assessment of interventions: phase I of the GUIDE trial. J Am Coll 21:134 A (Abst)
41. Stone GW, Hodgson JM, St Goar FG, et al. (1997) Improved procedural results of coronary angioplasty with intravascular ultrasound-guided balloon sizing. The CLOUT pilot trial. Circulation 95:2044–2052
42. The GUIDE Trial Investigators (1996) IVUS-determined predictors of restenosis in PTCA and DCA: Final report from the GUIDE trial, Phase 2. J Am Coll Cardiol 27:156 A (Abst)
43. Hosokawa H, Suzuki T, Ueno K, et al. (1996) Clinical and angiographic follow-up of adjunctive balloon angioplasty following coronary atherectomy study (ABACAS). Circulation 94:I-318 (Abst)
44. Simonton CA, Leon MB, Baim DS, et al. (1998) Optimal directional coronary atherectomy. Results of the Optimal Atherectomy Restenosis Study. Circulation 97:332–339
45. Nakamura S, Colombo A, Gaglione A, et al. (1994) Intracoronary ultrasound observations during stent implantation. Circulation 89:2026–2034
46. Colombo A, Hall P, Nakamura S, et al. (1995) Intracoronary stenting without anticoagulation accomplished with intravascular ultrasound guidance. Circulation 91:1676–1688
47. Karrillon GJ, Morice MC, Benveniste E, et al. (1996) Intracoronary stent implantation without ultrasound guidance and with replacement of conventional anticoagulation by antiplatelet therapy. 30-day clinical outcome of the French multicenter registry. Circulation 94:1518–1527
48. Goods CM, Al-Shaibi KF, Yadav SS, et al. (1996) Utilization of the coronary balloon-expandable coil stent without anticoagulation or intravascular ultrasound. Circulation 93:1803–1808

49. Bilodeau L, Doucet S, Tardif JC, et al. (1996) Can quantitative coronary analysis replace intravascular ultrasound to assess optimal stent deployment. J Am Coll Cardiol 27:305 A (Abst)
50. de Jaegere P, Mudra H, Almagor Y, et al. (1996) In-hospital and 1-month clinical results of an international study testing the concept of IVUS guided optimized stent expansion alleviating the need of systemic anticoagulation. J Am Coll Cardiol 27:137 A (Abst)
51. Mintz GS, Popma JJ, Pichard AD, et al. (1996) Arterial remodeling after coronary angioplasty. A serial intravascular ultrasound study. Circulation 94:35–43
52. Tardif JC, Côté G, Lespérance J, et al. (1997) Effect of probucol on vascular remodeling and tissue hyperplasia after coronary angioplasty: Intravascular ultrasound results from the MVP randomized trial. Circulation 96:I-154 (Abst)
53. Di Mario C, Gil R, Camenzind E, et al. (1995) Quantitative assessment with intra-coronary ultrasound of the mechanisms of restenosis after percutaneous transluminal coronary angioplasty and directional coronary atherectomy. Am J Cardiol 75:772–777
54. Hoffmann R, Mintz GS, Dussaillant GR, et al. (1996) Patterns and mechanisms of in-stent restenosis. A serial intravascular ultrasound study. Circulation 94:1247–1254
55. Libby P, Ganz P (1997) Restenosis revisited. New targets, new therapies. N Engl J Med 337:418–419
56. Tardif JC, Côté G, Lespérance J, et al. (1997) Probucol and multivitamins in the prevention of restenosis after coronary angioplasty. N Engl J Med 337:365–372
57. Tierstein PS, Massullo V, Jani S, et al. (1997) Catheter-based radiotherapy to inhibit restenosis after coronary stenting. N Engl J Med 336:1697–1703
58. Bonan R, Arsenault A, Tardif JC, et al. (1997) Beta Energy Restenosis Trial, Canadian arm. Circulation 96:I-219 (Abst)
59. Takagi T, Yoshida K, Akasaka T, et al. (1997) Intravascular ultrasound analysis of reduction in progression of coronary narrowing by treatment with pravastatin. Am J Cardiol 79:1673–1676
60. Brown G, Albers JJ, Fisher LD, et al. (1990) Regression of coronary artery disease as a result of intensive lipid-lowering therapy in men with high levels of apolipoprotein B. N Engl J Med 323:1289–1298
61. Evans JL, Ng KH, Wiet SG, et al. (1996) Accurate three-dimensional reconstruction of intravascular ultrasound data. Circulation 93:567–576
62. Roelandt JRTC, di Mario C, Pandian NG, et al. (1994) Three-dimensional reconstruction of intracoronary ultrasound images. Rationale, approaches, problems, and directions. Circulation 90:1044–1055

Non-Antithrombotic Treatment of Acute Coronary Syndromes: Role of Beta-Blockers, Calcium Channel Blockers, and Nitrates

X. Bosch

Introduction

Beta-blockers, calcium channel blockers, and nitrates are anti-ischemic agents with proven efficacy in relieving angina in patients with coronary artery disease. Although these agents differ in their mechanisms of action, they increase coronary blood flow and reduce myocardial oxygen demand. These effects can be expected to be of benefit in acute coronary syndromes like unstable angina (UA) and acute myocardial infarction (AMI). However, relieving pain is only a minor goal in the treatment of unstable coronary syndromes, the major goals being the treatment of myocardial ischemia, the preservation of left ventricular function, and the improvement of prognosis.

In this chapter we summarize the extent of the available evidence on the effect of these agents on prognosis, especially the occurrence of myocardial infarction and mortality, in patients with AMI and UA.

Beta-Blockers

Beta-blockers reduce heart rate, blood pressure, and contractility, and, thus, reduce myocardial oxygen consumption. They also induce coronary blood flow redistribution from the epicardium to the endocardium, and inhibit cate-cholamine-induced lipolysis during acute ischemia reducing circulating free fatty acids. In animal models, they have proved to reduce infarct size and increase the threshold for ventricular fibrillation. On the other side, the negative inotropic and chronotropic effect may be harmful during acute ischemia.

Acute Myocardial Infarction

Beta-blockers may be administered early during prolonged ischemia with the aim to prevent myocardial infarction, decrease the intensity of pain and the incidence of ventricular arrhythmias, limit the extent of the infarct size, prevent reinfarction, and increase survival. They also can be administered orally after the infarction with the aim of preventing reinfarction and sudden death.

Early Treatment

As with thrombolytic treatment, any drug administered during the acute phase of myocardial infarction is likely to obtain the greatest benefit when administered during the first 6–12 h. Thus, to obtain immediate beta blockade, these drugs should be administered intravenously. The two largest studies performed in this setting were the ISIS-1 [1] and the MIAMI [2] trials. The greatest experience with beta-blockers in the early hours of AMI has been obtained with propranolol, atenolol and metoprolol.

Prevention of Definite Myocardial Infarction
In five trials [1, 3–6], specific data are available on 4706 patients without definite ECG evidence of AMI at the time of treatment allocation. Overall, 28.8% of patients randomized to treatment with beta-blockers developed an AMI compared to 31.6% of control patients, resulting in a 13% risk reduction ($p<0.05$) [7].

Limitation of Infarct Size
Trials on reduction of infarct size have the limitation of the difficulty of measuring this important outcome in patients. However, this limitation is expected to be equally distributed in active and control groups in randomized studies. Ten trials have studied this effect on a total of 2639 patients by measuring serum enzyme levels [4, 5, 10–15]. Eight of them found a statistical significant reduction on enzyme release favoring beta-blockade. Overall, a reduction of 20% in infarct size ($p<0.01$) was obtained by early intravenous beta-blockade [7].

Reinfarction
The incidence of reinfarction during the hospital stay is available on 23700 patients [7]. In the beta-blocker treated group, 327 of 11823 patients (2.8%) suffered a reinfarction compared to 404 of 11858 patients (3.4%) in the control group, resulting in a risk reduction of 20%, with a 95% confidence interval of 7–31%, $p<0.02$ (Fig. 1). In the thrombolytic era, only one trial (TIMI IIb) studied the effects of beta-blockers on the incidence of reinfarction [16]. In this study, reinfarction was reduced from 5.1% to 2.7% ($p=0.02$), postinfarction angina decreased from 24.1% to 18.8% ($p=0.02$), and intracranial bleeding was reduced from 0.8% to 0% ($p=0.03$).

Mortality
In ISIS-1 [1], mortality was reduced from 4.6% to 3.9% ($p<0.04$) during hospitalization, while in the MIAMI trial [2] no significant difference was observed in spite of obtaining the same degree of relative risk reduction (13%). When the results of these two large randomized trials are combined with the results obtained in 28 small trials [7], the mortality reduction in the beta-blocker treated group is of 13%, with a 95% confidence interval from 3% to 23% ($p<0.02$; Fig. 1). The mechanism by which beta-blockers reduce mortality is multifactorial. It has been shown in 27 trials [4, 17, 18] that beta-blockade reduces the incidence of ventricular fibrillation by 15%±7%, from 2.6% to 2.2% ($p<0.05$). Fur-

Early ß-Blockade and Short-term Prognosis
Pooled Data of 32 Trials on 29,200 patients

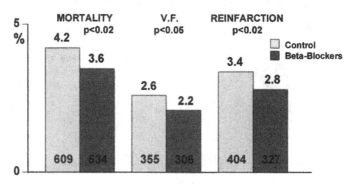

Fig. 1. Effect of the administration of intravenous beta-blockers during the early hours of acute myocardial infarction on in-hospital mortality and reinfarction. *Bottom of bars* number of patients with events

thermore, a retrospective analysis of ISIS-1 [19] and one metoprolol trial [20] has shown that the early benefit was obtained mostly by decreasing myocardial rupture.

Long-Term Treatment

After the acute phase of an AMI, there is still a potential for benefit from beta-blockade to prevent reinfarction and sudden death. Eighteen trials studying 20,300 patients have been performed starting oral beta-blockers several days after AMI, 8 other trials on 3900 patients in which beta-blockade was started during the early hours, were continued on a long term basis.

Mortality

The largest and most significant trials were the Norwegian timolol trial [21], the BHAT propranolol trial [22], and the Metoprolol trials [20, 23]. In all of these trials a benefit or a positive trend were observed with both cardioselective and non-selective agents. Overall, in the beta-blockade arm of these trials mortality occurred in 934 of 12,438 patients (7.5%) compared to 1124 of 11,832 patients (9.5%) in the control groups (Fig. 2). This benefit represents a 23% reduction in the odds of death ($p<0.0001$), with a 95% CI ranging from 16% to 30%. It is important to note that the benefit has been observed in all subgroups analyzed, although the greater benefit were observed in the BHAT, MIAMI and timolol trials, in patients with a history of heart failure [2, 24]. Another issue is if beta-blockade is also beneficial when a beta-blocker with ISA effect is administered. Recently, it has been shown that the mortality reduction is of 27% with agents without ISA and of 17% for agents with ISA. Thus, although a less pronounced effect is

Effect of long-term Beta-Blockade After AMI.
Pooled Data of 26 Trials on 24,200 pts.

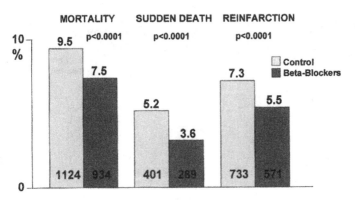

Fig. 2. Effect of the administration of oral beta-blockers after the acute phase of myocardial infarction on long-term mortality and reinfarction. *Bottom of bars* number of patients with events

observed with those agents, there is still a beneficial effect. Subgroup analysis has also shown that the mortality reduction is obtained mostly by reducing sudden death (32%±5%), but non-sudden death is also reduced (12%±7%).

Reinfarction
Data on reinfarction is available on 20,400 patients [1]. Overall, this event was reduced from 7.3% to 5.5%, resulting in a 27% risk reduction, with a 95% confidence interval ranging from 18% to 35%, $p<0.0001$ (Fig. 2).

Use of Beta-Blockers in AMI in the Real World

Despite the demonstrated efficacy of beta-blockers during the early hours of AMI and at long-term, physicians had been reluctant for many years to prescribe these drugs to most of the patients with infarctions. The reasons include the fear to adverse effects, both cardiac (heart failure, AV block), and non-cardiac (bronchospasm, fatigue, impotence). Furthermore, many physicians feel that the number of patients needed to be treated to save one live is to high, that no sufficient subgroup analysis has been performed to stratify high risk patients that could most benefit from prophylactic treatment, and, finally, that the results of old studies do not apply to the actual era of thrombolysis, antiplatelet drugs, risk stratification and coronary intervention. As a result, only one third of the patients in the United States and in Spain are being treated with beta-blockers and two thirds in Europe (Fig. 3). Furthermore, patients that could potentially benefit most from long-term beta-blockade, i.e. those with diabetes, prior heart failure or with left ventricular dysfunction, are less frequently treated than patients without these characteristics [25].

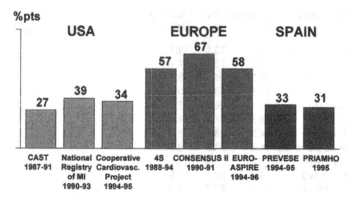

Fig. 3. Use of beta-blockers after myocardial infarction in United States and Europe in different studies and registries performed from 1987 to 1996

Adverse Effects

Heart failure is the most feared adverse effect in patients with AMI treated with beta-blockers. However, in selected patients in which this condition was not present at the time of randomization, the incidence of heart failure was similar in patients on beta-blockers compared with the control groups in acute phase trials (17.5% versus 16.8%, NS), and only slightly higher in long term trials (5.9% versus 5.4%, $p<0.05$). The results on A-V block are similar (3.1% versus 2.9%), but they only apply to patients without bradycardia or conduction disturbances at baseline.

Results in the Thrombolytic Era

All but the above mentioned TIMI II-b trial, on beta-blockers in patients with AMI, were performed in the pre-thrombolytic era in patients with higher mortality risk than patients treated nowadays. Furthermore, in those trials, patients in which beta-blockers showed to have a greater benefit, i.e., those with left ventricular dysfunction or prior heart failure, were not taking ACE inhibitors, medication that has proved to reduce mortality in this patient population. However, in the SAVE study [26], beta-blocker use was associated with a 30% reduction in the risk of cardiovascular death (95% CI 12% to 44%), and a 21% reduction of development of heart failure (95% CI 3% to 36%). Furthermore, in a recent survey of 201,752 postinfarction patients performed in the United States during 1994–1995 [25], the use of beta-blockers was associated with a 40% reduction in mortality at 2 years, from 23.9% to 14.4% (Fig. 4). Among patients that were treated with thrombolytic agents, mortality was reduced from 19.6% to 11.8%, resulting in a absolute risk reduction of 7.8 and a relative risk reduction of 40% (95% CI from 37% to 43%). It is to note that, in this registry, beta-blockade was beneficial in all subgroups of patients including those with uncomplicated infarctions and those with chronic obstructive pulmonary disease.

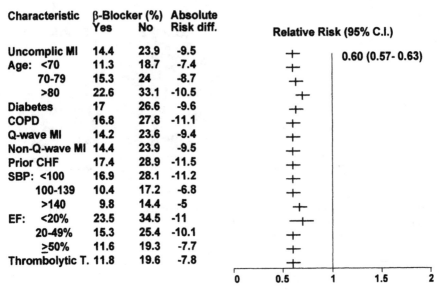

Characteristic	β-Blocker (%) Yes	No	Absolute Risk diff.
Uncomplic MI	14.4	23.9	-9.5
Age: <70	11.3	18.7	-7.4
70-79	15.3	24	-8.7
>80	22.6	33.1	-10.5
Diabetes	17	26.6	-9.6
COPD	16.8	27.8	-11.1
Q-wave MI	14.2	23.6	-9.4
Non-Q-wave MI	14.4	23.9	-9.5
Prior CHF	17.4	28.9	-11.5
SBP: <100	16.9	28.1	-11.2
100-139	10.4	17.2	-6.8
>140	9.8	14.4	-5
EF: <20%	23.5	34.5	-11
20-49%	15.3	25.4	-10.1
≥50%	11.6	19.3	-7.7
Thrombolytic T.	11.8	19.6	-7.8

Relative Risk (95% C.I.)   0.60 (0.57- 0.63)

Fig. 4. Adjusted risk and relative risk of death after myocardial infarction according to the administration of beta-blockers at the time of hospital discharge in different subgroup of patients. Data from the Cooperative Cardiovascular Project [25]. A 40% decrease in the risk of death was observed with small variations between subgroups, including patients with uncomplicated infarcts and those who were treated with thrombolytics. The higher absolute benefit was observed in older patients, diabetics, those with chronic obstructive pulmonary disease, and those with prior heart failure or with left ventricular dysfunction. *CHF* Cardiac heart failure; *C.I.* confidence intervals; *COPD* chronic obstructive pulmonary disease; *EF* ejection fraction; *MI* myocardial infarction; *SBP* systolic blood pressure

Thus it seems clear that the benefit obtained by the use of beta-blockers is maintained in the thrombolytic era, although direct, prospective comparisons have not been performed. To obviate this important limitation, currently, the COMET study is comparing the effect of Carvedilol versus Metoprolol in patients with AMI, while the CAPRICORN study is analyzing the effect of Carvedilol in patients with AMI and left ventricular dysfunction (Ejection Fraction lower than 40%) who are being treated with ACE inhibitors. The results of both studies are expected to be reported during year 2000.

Unstable Angina

Contrary to the large body of evidence existing with the use of beta-blockers in patients with AMI, only two randomized trials have been performed in patients with Unstable Angina. In the HINT trial [27], 79 patients were randomized to be treated with metoprolol and 84 with placebo. AMI occurred in 13 patients in each group and AMI or recurrent ischemia in 22 patients (28%) in the metoprolol group compared to 31 patients (37%) in the placebo group. In another trial, in which propranolol or identical placebo were added to calcium blockers or nitrates

[28], 6 of 42 patients in the beta-blocker group, compared to 3 of 39 patients in the placebo group, had an AMI. However, the number of ischemic episodes were significantly lower in the propranolol group.

Finally, in the Cooperative Cardiovascular Project [25], patients with non-Q wave infarctions had the same degree of benefit from beta-blockade than patients with Q wave MI.

Calcium Channel Blockers

Most studies have been performed using nifedipine, diltiazem and verapamil. All of them induce coronary vasodilation, increase oxygen supply to the myocardium, and decrease myocardial oxygen consumption. Furthermore, they may decrease reperfusion injury and had proven to limit infarct size in experimental models of ischemia and reperfusion.

Acute Myocardial Infarction

Data are available on 19,600 patients that were randomized to treatment to calcium channel blockers or placebo in 23 controlled trials in patients with AMI [29]. In 16 trials with a total of 11100 patients, treatment was started during the acute phase, and continued only during hospitalization in 6300 patients and long term in 4800. Late therapy was studied in four trials of 8400 patients.

Early Treatment

Nifedipine
In one study of 4491 patients [30], mortality was of 6.7% in the nifedipine group versus 6.3% in the placebo group (NS), while the incidence of reinfarction was 1.5% versus 2.2% respectively (NS). The SPRINT-II trial [31] was stopped when 1358 patients were randomized because of a trend toward increased mortality in the active treatment group. At that time, mortality was of 15% in the nifedipine group versus 13% in the control group, while the incidence of definite myocardial infarction was of 84% versus 87%, NS.

Diltiazem
Three trials have studied the effect of diltiazem on infarct size. While in two, non significant differences were observed, the last one found a significant increase in infarct size in the diltiazem group [32]. In one study on non-Q wave AMI in which treatment was started 24–72 h after hospital admission and continued for 2 weeks [33], the incidence of reinfarction was marginally lower in patients randomized to diltiazem ($2p=0.06$).

Verapamil
Intravenous followed by high dose oral verapamil (120 mg TID) was administered in the DAVIT-I study [34] in which 3498 patients were randomized. Definite AMI

was observed in the same proportion (42%) of patients taking verapamil or place-bo. In 13 small trials in which 1800 patients were evaluated using nifedipine or verapamil, 60.8% of those treated with calcium channel blockers developed an AMI compared to 61.4% of controls [37]. After all this high amount of evidence, it seems clear that prophylactic administration of calcium channel blockers during the early hours of an AMI do not prevent the development of AMI or rein-farction, and does not seem to limit infarct size or decrease acute mortality either.

Long-Term Treatment

Nifedipine
No differences in reinfarction or mortality were found in the SPRINT-1 trial [35], in which 2276 patients were studied. The SPRINT-II trial [31] was stopped pre-maturely because of a trend to higher mortality in the nifedipine group.

Diltiazem
In the MDPIT trial [36], 2466 patients were randomized. At 2 years mortality was 13.5% in both active and control groups while reinfarction occurred in 8% of patients treated with diltiazem compared to 9.4% of patients of the control group (NS). In a retrospective subgroup analysis the incidence of heart failure and mor-tality was observed to be significantly higher in patients with prior pulmonary congestion or left ventricular dysfunction who were on diltiazem, while a trend to lower mortality was observed in patients on diltiazem without these characteris-tics.

Verapamil
In the DAVIT-I trial [34], after a 6-months follow-up, there were 50 reinfarctions in the group treated with verapamil versus 60 in the placebo group. Mortality occurred in 8.6% and 8.4% respectively. In DAVIT-II [37], mortality was 10.8% in the verapamil group and 13.3% in the placebo group (NS), and reinfarction was observed in 9.6% and 11.9% of patients in each group respectively (NS).

Overall Effects

Overall, no beneficial effects have been observed with the prophylactic adminis-tration of calcium channel blockers in patients with AMI, both during the acute phase and at long term (Fig. 5). In fact, a significant trend to higher mortality and reinfarction rates have been observed with the use of nifedipine when all trials with calcium channel blockers have been combined [29, 38]. The results obtained with diltiazem and verapamil show a non-significant trend to lower reinfarction rates. When all the studies with these two drugs are combined, a sig-nificant 20% reduction in the incidence of reinfarction is observed ($p<0.01$), with a 95% confidence interval ranging from 6% to 33% (Fig. 5). It seems, there-fore, that calcium channel blockers that decrease heart rate may be of benefit in patients with AMI although less marked than the effect obtained with beta-blockers. Nifedipine, however, induce a catecholamine response, increase heart rate and tend to increase mortality and reinfarction. These results are consistent

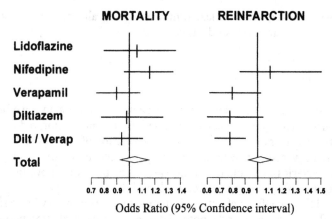

Fig. 5. Odds ratios and 95% confidence intervals for death and reinfarction in patients treated with calcium channel blockers during and after myocardial infarction [37]

with the higher mortality found in trials where nifedipine or nicardipine were administered in patients with stable angina [39, 40]. Such deleterious effects have not been observed, however, in patients treated with long-acting preparations of nifedipine. Recently, the results of the NICOLE study have been orally reported. In this trial in which nisoldipine was administered in patients with AMI, no significant differences have been observed among patients treated with nisoldipine or placebo.

Unstable Angina

Only nifedipine and diltiazem have been studied in patients with the syndrome of unstable angina/non-Q wave MI. In the HINT trial [27], the incidence of AMI or recurrent ischemia 48 h after hospital admission was of 47.2% in the nifedipine group compared to 36.9% in the placebo group (NS). This trend toward a worst prognosis with the administration of nifedipine, was not observed with the concomitant use of metoprolol. In another study [41], no differences on prognosis were observed between nifedipine and placebo, while other studies comparing nifedipine [42] or diltiazem [43] with beta-blockers did not find differences in the incidence of recurrent ischemia.

In patients with non-Q wave AMI, diltiazem reduced the incidence of reinfarction from 9.3% to 5.2% ($2p=0.06$), while the mortality rate was of 3.8% with diltiazem and 3.1% with placebo (NS) [33]. It is to note that two thirds of the patients in this study were taking concomitant beta-blockers. In the MDPIT trial [36], 634 patients with non-Q wave AMI were randomized and a trend to lower reinfarctions in the diltiazem group were observed (8.4% compared to 10.9%, NS). Similar data have been observed in the DAVIT-II trial [37].

Overall, the results obtained in patients with unstable angina/non-Q wave MI indicate that short-acting nifedipine seems to be detrimental when given without a beta-blocker, while diltiazem may be a good alternative to beta-blockers when these agents are contraindicated.

Nitrates

Nitrates induce vascular muscle relaxation resulting in vasodilation of veins, arteries, arterioles and collateral circulation. Venodilation reduces venous return to the heart, and, thus, reduces preload. Dilation of arteries and arterioles reduces systemic vascular resistance resulting in a decrease of afterload. Dilation of coronary arteries and collaterals increase coronary blood flow. In addition, nitrates improve subendocardial coronary blood flow.

All this beneficial effects on ischemic myocardium may be counterbalanced by a reflex tachycardia, and a potential of myocardial perfusion pressure decrease as a result of their effect on blood pressure. This is specially important in patients with right ventricular infarction.

In spite of such a potential for a beneficial effect on prognosis, only a few randomized controlled trials have been performed using nitrates in patients with AMI, and none in patients with unstable angina.

Acute Myocardial Infarction

Three trials have been performed using nitroprusside, seven using intravenous nitroglycerin, and five with oral nitrates.

Early Intravenous Treatment

Nitroprusside
In one trial on 328 patients, nitroprusside significantly reduced mortality from 12% to 6%, $p<0.05$ [44]. In another trial performed on 812 patients [45], only a trend to fewer deaths was observed (17% compared to 19%, NS). Finally, a small trial on 50 high risk patients [46] showed also a trend to fewer deaths among patients allocated to active treatment (28% versus 36%, NS). Overall, in these three trials mortality was 85 of 595 (14.3%) in patients randomized to nitroprusside, compared to 106 of 595 (17.8%) in controls (NS) [47].

Nitroglycerin
Until recently, all the trials on nitroglycerin were performed with small populations, and showed a trend to lower mortality rate [47]. In the GISSI-3 trial [49], 19,394 patients were randomized to intravenous nitroglycerin for 24 h followed by transdermal nitroglycerin for 6 weeks. There was a non-significant 6% decrease in mortality, from 6.9% to 6.5%. However, intravenous nitroglycerin did significantly decrease the incidence of postinfaction angina ($p=0.03$) and cardiogenic shock ($p<0.01$).

Long-Term Treatment

In ISIS-4 [50], 58,050 patients were randomized to oral slow-release isosorbide mononitrate or placebo within the first 24 h. The one-month results showed no difference in mortality in the nitrate group (7.34%) compared to the control group (7.54%). Although postinfarction angina occurred less frequently in patients on nitrates, the incidence of cardiogenic shock was similar. In the GISSI-3 [49], patients randomized to intravenous nitroglycerin were treated during 6 weeks with transdermal nitroglycerin. No differences in mortality were observed among the active or the control group.

It is to note, that both in GISSI-3 and ISIS-4, 60% of the patients not allocated to nitrates received that therapy at admission, mostly as intravenous nitroglycerin. This may have obscured a possible benefit of nitrates in the early hours of AMI. The results are more convincing for long-term oral nitrate or transdermal nitroglycerin therapy since in GISSI-3, only 11% of the controls received nitrate therapy for more than 5 days.

A meta-analysis of all reported studies on the use of nitrates in AMI [50] found a significant 5.5% reduction in mortality, which means that we have to treat 1000 patients to save 4 lives (Fig. 6).

Unstable Angina

No randomized controlled trials have been performed to evaluate the effects of nitrates on the prognosis of patients with Unstable Angina. In a review of nine uncontrolled trials on a total of 280 patients [51] treated with intravenous nitroglycerin, no definite conclusion could be reached.

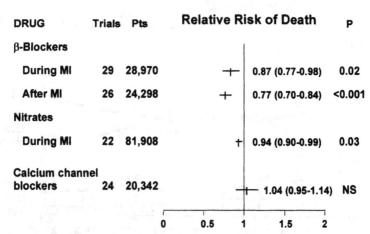

Fig. 6. Meta-analyses of randomized trials of antianginal therapy administered during and after myocardial infarction

Actual Use of Beta-Blockers, Calcium Channel Blockers and Nitrates in Patients with Myocardial Infarction

Despite the evidence favoring early and late administration of beta-blockers in patients with AMI, only 36%–42% of the 240,989 patients enrolled in the National Registry of Myocardial Infarction in the United States from 1990 to 1993 received such therapy [30]. On the other side, despite their lack of benefit in randomized trials, calcium channel blockers were prescribed in 30%–40% of the patients. In Spain, data from the PRIAMHO study, a national registry of 33 Coronary Care Units, show that during the years 1994–1997, i.v. nitroglycerin has been administered to 70% of the patients in a regular manner, while the use of oral nitrates has decreased from 36% of the patients at the end of 1994 to 26% in 1997 (Fig. 7). During the same period, the administration of beta-blockers during the acute phase increased from 24% to 40% while the use of calcium channel blockers decreased from 11% to 6.5% for diltiazem, and from less than 5% to 1–2% for nifedipine and verapamil.

Conclusions

During acute myocardial infarction, beta-blockers should be administered intravenously in addition to aspirin and thrombolytic therapy, if no contraindications exists. Late treatment with oral beta-blockers improves the prognosis of patients with AMI, specially in those with prior heart failure. Since no prospective con-

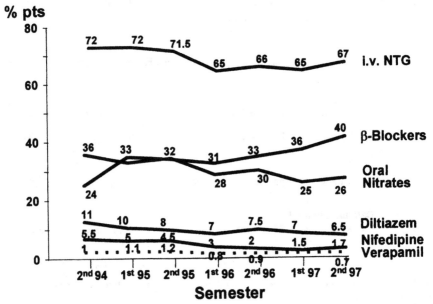

Fig. 7. Use of beta-blockers, calcium channel blockers and nitrates in a representative sample of 33 coronary care units in Spain from 1994 to 1997. Data from the PRIAMHO Registry

trolled studies have been performed on the effects of beta-blockers in patients treated with thrombolytics and antiplatelet drugs that are treated with ACE inhibitors, trials that are currently studying the effects of beta-blockers in this situation are specially awaited.

Calcium channel blockers should not be given routinely to prevent complications, but only if ischemic complications occur, and only if contraindications exists for the use of beta-blockers; In this case, diltiazem or verapamil should be used.

Intravenous nitroglycerin may be useful during the first 24 h in certain subgroup of patients like those with high blood pressure, those with persistent chest pain, those with large infarcts or with heart failure, provided that no hypotension or tachycardia is induced. Prophylactic treatment with oral nitrates is not indicated in patients with AMI.

Although the amount of evidence is scarce in patients with unstable angina, beta-blockers are the drugs of choice in addition to antiplatelet drugs and heparin. Calcium channel blockers should be used only if contraindications to beta blockers exists or in addition to these drugs. Nifedipine should be administered only with concomitant beta-blockade. Nitrates, and specially intravenous nitroglycerin, are very effective in relieving pain and preventing recurrent ischemia and is currently used during the first 24 h, and when symptoms recur before revascularization strategies can be performed.

Acknowledgements. This article was supported in part with a grant from Fondo de Investigaciones Sanitarias FIS 98/0410, Spain.

References

1. ISIS-1 (First International Study of Infarct Survival) Collaborative Group (1986). Randomized trial of intravenous atenolol among 16,027 cases of suspected acute myocardial infarction. ISIS-1. Lancet 2:57–65.
2. The MIAMI trial research group (1985). Metoprolol in Acute Myocardial Infarction: (MIAMI). A randomized placebo-controlled international trial. Eur Heart J 6:199–226.
3. Norris RM, Sammel NL, Clarke E, Smith WM (1978). Protective effect of propranolol in threatened myocardial infarction. Lancet 2:907–909.
4. Yusuf S, Sleight P, Rossi PRF, et al. (1983). Reduction in infarct size, arrhythmias, chest pain, and morbidity by early intravenous beta-blockade in suspected acute myocardial infarction. Circulation 67:32–41.
5. Herlitz J, Emanuelsson H, Swedberg K, et al. (1984). Göteborg Metoprolol Trial. Enzyme-estimated infarct size. Am J Cardiol 53:15D-21D, 1984.
6. The MIAMI Trial Research Group (1985). Development of myocardial infarction. Am J Cardiol 56:23G-26G.
7. Hennekens CH, Albert CM, Godfried SL, Gaziano JM, Buring JE (1996). Adjunctive drug therapy of acute myocardial infarction. Evidence from clinical trials. N Engl J Med 335:1660-67
8. Peter T, Norris RM, Clarke DE, et al. (1978). Reduction of enzyme levels by propranolol after acute myocardial infarction. Circulation 57:1091–1095.
9. Norris RM, Sammel NL, Clarke DE, et al. (1980). Treatment of acute myocardial infarction with propranolol: Further studies on enzyme appearance and subsequent left ventricular function in treated and control patients with developing infarcts. Br Heart J 43:617–622.

10. Lloyd EA, Gordon GD, Mabin TA, et al. (1982). Intravenous sotalol in acute myocardial infarction. Circulation 2 (suppl):983.

11. Boyle DM, Barber JM, McIlmoyle EL, et al. (1983). Effect estimation of infarct size. Br Heart J 49:229-233.

12. International Collaborative Study Group (1984). Reduction of infarct size with the early use of timolol in acute myocardial infarction. N Engl J Med 310:9-15.

13. Roberts R, Croft C, Gold HK, et al. (1984). Effect of propranolol on myocardial infarct size in a randomized blinded multicenter trial. N Engl J Med 311:218-225.

14. The MIAMI Trial Research Group (1985). Enzymatic estimation of infarct size. Am J Cardiol 56:27G-29G.

15. Roque R, Amuchastegui LM, Lopez Morillos MA, et al. (1986). Beneficial effects of timolol on infarct size and late ventricular tachycardia in patients with acute myocardial infarction. Circulation 76:610-617.

16. Roberts R, Rogers WJ, Mueller HS, et al. (1991): Immediate versus deferred β-blockade following thrombolytic therapy in patients with acute myocardial infarction. Results of the Thrombolysis in Myocardial Infarction (TIMI) II-B Study. Circulation 83:422-437.

17. Rydén L, Arniego R, Arnman KI, et al. (1983). A double-blind trial of metoprolol in acute myocardial infarction: Effects on ventricular tachycardia. N Engl J Med 308:614-618.

18. Norris RM, Barnaby P, Brown MA, et al. (1984). Prevention of ventricular fibrillation during acute myocardial infarction by intravenous propranolol. Lancet 2:883-886.

19. ISIS-1 (First International Study of Infarct Survival) Collaborative Group (1988). Possible mechanisms for the early mortality reduction produced by beta-blockade started early in acute myocardial infarction. Lancet 1:921-923.

20. Hjalmarson A, Elmfeldt D, Herlitz J, et al. (1981). Effect on mortality of metoprolol in acute myocardial infarction: A double-blind randomised trial. Lancet 2:823-827, 1981.

21. Norwegian Multicenter Study Group (1981). Timolol-induced reduction in mortality and reinfarction in patients surviving acute myocardial infarction. N Engl J Med 304:801-807, 1981.

22. Beta-Blocker Heart Attack Trial Research Group (1982). A randomized trial of propranolol in patients with acute myocardial infarction. I. Mortality results. JAMA 247:1707-1714, 1982.

23. Salathia KS, Barber JM, McIlmoyle EL, et al. (1985). Very early intervention with metoprolol in suspected acute myocardial infarction. Eur Heart J 6:190-198, 1985.

24. Chadda K, Goldstein S, Byington R, Curb JD (1986). Effect of propranolol after myocardial infarction in patients with congestive heart failure. Circulation 73:503-510.

25. Gottlieb SS, McCarter RJ, Vogel RA (1998). Effect of beta-blockade on mortality among high-risk and low-risk patients after myocardial infarction. N Engl J Med 1998;339:489-97.

26. Vantrimpont P, Rouleau JL, Wun CC, Ciampi A, Klein M, Sussex B et al. (1997). Additive beneficial effects of beta-blockers to angiotensin-converting enzyme inhibitors in the survival and ventricular enlargement (SAVE) study. J Am Coll Cardiol 29:229-36.

27. Holland Interuniversity Nifedipine/Metoprolol Trial (HINT) Research Group (1986). Early treatment of unstable angina in the coronary care unit: A randomized, double-blind placebo controlled comparison of recurrent ischemia in patients treated with nifedipine or metoprolol or both. Br Heart J 56:400-413.

28. Gottlieb SO, Weisfeldt MD, Ouyang P, et al. (1986). Effect of the addiction of propranolol to therapy with nifedipine for unstable angina pectoris: A randomized double-blind, placebo controlled trial. Circulation 73:331-337.

29. Held PH, Yusuf S, Furberg CD (1989). Calcium channel blockers in acute myocardial infarction and unstable angina: An overview. Br Med J 299:1187-1192.

30. Wilcox RG, Hampton JR, Banks DC, et al. (1986). Trial of early nifedipine in acute myocardial infarction: The TRENT study. Br Med J 293:1204.

31. SPRINT Study Group (1988). The secondary prevention re-infarction Israeli nifedipine trial (SPRINT) II: design and methods, results. Eur Heart J 9 (suppl 1):350.

32. Bartels L, Remme W, Wiesfeld A, van der Laarse A (1992). High-dose intravenous diltiazem increases infarct size in acute, uncomplicated myocardial infarction. A placebo-controlled study. J Am Coll Cardiol 19:381.

33. Gibson RS, Boden WE, Théroux P, et al. (1986). Diltiazem and reinfarction in patients with non-Q wave myocardial infarction. N Engl J Med 315:423.

34. Danish Study Group on Verapamil in Myocardial Infarction (1984). Verapamil in acute myocardial infarction. Eur Heart J 5:516.

35. The Israeli SPRINT Study Group (1988). Secondary prevention reinfarction Israeli nifedipine trial (SPRINT). A randomized intervention trial of nifedipine in patients with acute myocardial infarction. Eur Heart J 9:354–364.

36. The Multicenter Diltiazem Postinfarction Trial Research Group (1988). The effect of diltiazem on mortality and reinfarction after myocardial infarction. N Engl J Med 319:385–392.

37. The Danish Study Group on Verapamil in Myocardial Infarction (1990) Secondary prevention with verapamil after myocardial infarction. Am J Cardiol 66:331–401.

38. Yusuf S, Held P, Furberg C (1991). Update of effects of calcium antagonists in myocardial infarction or angina in light of the Second Danish Verapamil Infarction Trial (DAVIT-II) and other recent studies. Am J Cardiol 67:1295–1297.

39. Lichtlen PR, Hugenholtz PG, Rafflenbeul W, Hecker H, Jost S, Deckers JW (1990). On behalf of the INTACT group investigators. Lancet 335:1109–1113.

40. Waters D, Lespérance J, Francetich M, et al. (1990). A controlled clinical trial to assess the effect of a calcium channel blocker on the progression of coronary atherosclerosis. Circulation 82:!940–1953.

41. Gerstenblith G, Ouyang P, Achuff SC, et al. (1982). Nifedipine in unstable angina. A double-blind, randomized trial. N Engl J Med 306:885–889.

42. Muller JE, Turi ZG, Pearle DL, et al. (1984). Nifedipine and conventional therapy for unstable angina pectoris: A randomized, double-blind comparison. Circulation 69:728–739.

43. Théroux PO, Taeymans Y, Morissette D, Bosch X, Pelletier GB, Waters DD (1985). A randomized study comparing propranolol and diltiazem in the treatment of unstable angina. J Am Coll Cardiol 5:717–722.

44. Durrer JD, Lie KI, Van Capelle FJL, Durrer D (1982). Effect of sodium nitroprusside on mortality in acute myocardial infarction. N Engl J Med 306:1121–1128.

45. Cohn JN, Franciosa JA, Francis GS, et al. (1982). Effect of short-term infusion of sodium nitroprusside on mortality rate in acute myocardial infarction complicated by left ventricular failure. Results of a Veterans Administration Cooperative Study. N Engl J Med 306:1129–1135.

46. Hockings BEF, Cope GD, Clarke GM, Taylor RR (1981). Randomized controlled trial of vasodilator therapy after myocardial infarction. Am J Cardiol 48:345–352, 1981.

47. Yusuf S, Collins R, MacMahon S, Peto R (1988). Effect of intravenous nitrates on mortality in acute myocardial infarction: An overview of the randomized trials. Lancet 1:1088–1092.

48. Jugdutt BI, Warnica JW (1988). Intravenous nitroglycerin therapy to limit myocardial infarct size, expansion, and complications. Effect of timing dosage, and infarct location. Circulation 78:906–919.

49. Gruppo Italiano per lo Studio della Sopravvivenza nell'Infarto Miocardico (1994). GISSI-3: effects of lisinopril and transdermal glyceryl trinitrate singly and together on 6-week mortality and ventricular function after acute myocardial infarction. Lancet 343:1115–22.

50. ISIS-4 (Fourth International Study of Infarct Survival) Collaborative Group (1995). ISIS-4: a randomised factorial trial assessing early oral captopril, oral mononitrate, and intravenous magnesium sulphate in 58050 patients with suspected acute myocardial infarction. Lancet 345:669–95.

51. Conti CR (1987). Use of nitrates in unstable angina pectoris. Am J Cardiol 60:31H-34H.

Coronary Circulation and Myocardial Ischaemia: Thrombolysis

P. Sleight

Introduction

The past 1–2 decades have seen a revolution in the treatment of myocardial infarction (MI), so that the case fatality of those who reach hospital has about halved [1]. This improvement has been related to several factors, but mainly to the timely dissolution of the culprit thrombus by thrombolytic drugs [2] or later by direct PTCA [3], and the enhancement of this process by inhibition of platelet aggregation by aspirin [4] and the newer more powerful IIb/IIIa receptor antagonists.

Although it seemed logical to use in addition a thrombin inhibitor such as Heparin or Hirudin, randomised trials have shown that the balance of risk and benefit when these are added to aspirin is rather marginal [5], except in the case of unstable angina where the thrombus is generally not totally occlusive. This paradox seems related partly to the difficulty in ensuring a safe and constant level of antithrombin activity with these drugs, and the danger of haemorrhage when this activity is too high, especially in the presence of thrombolytics.

In contrast, during the last few years we have seen a dramatic improvement in outcome with more effective antiplatelet agents, particularly in the setting of interventional cardiology [6]. It is likely that improved and orally acting antiplatelet agents will hold even greater promise in the medical treatment of the acute phase of MI, although their current high cost will be a deterrent to their wide use.

The Importance of Timely Treatment

In some ways the large benefits seen with these reperfusion strategies were unexpected. Animal models had shown that irreversible myocardial damage occurs after about 20 min of ischaemia and so it seemed unlikely that there would be much hope of intervention in man, given this time frame.

In retrospect, we now recognise that the animal models were flawed. First it is clear now that human coronary occlusion is a dynamic process with lysis (spontaneous) and coagulation occurring simultaneously. Maseri and his colleagues [7] used repeated angiography to show repeated opening and closing of the culprit lesion during thrombolysis, which was reflected in rapid ST segment shifts in the

ECG. We do not know whether this is related to coronary spasm or relaxation, or (more probably) to the dissolution and regrowth of largely platelet thrombi. This could also explain the surprisingly large benefits of early aspirin treatment in the initial phase of infarction. In ISIS-2 we were all very surprised that the benefit in patients given aspirin alone was almost as great as in those given streptokinase alone (Fig. 1 [4]).

Secondly, the presence of coronary collateral vessels in man, as a result of previous ischaemia, acts to prolong the period of myocardial necrosis in some patients, and these patients are very probably selectively enabled to survive long enough to call for help and arrive in hospital. Thus the patients who receive thrombolysis or PTCA and aspirin are a subgroup of all coronary occlusions.

Epidemiological studies have shown that only about 30% of all patients with MI reach hospital alive [1, 8]. The majority die outside hospital, many of them suddenly, before the possibility of receiving medical or paramedical help.

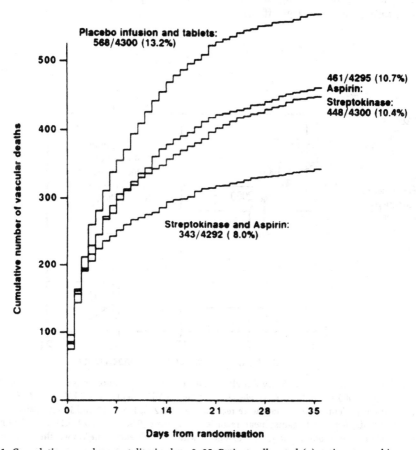

Fig. 1. Cumulative vascular mortality in days 0–35. Patients allocated (a) active streptokinase only, (b) active aspirin only, (c) both active treatments, and (d) neither. (With permission from [4])

Nevertheless overviews of both fibrinolytic and mechanical reperfusion have clearly shown a steep decline in benefit with each hour which passes from the onset of pain, approaching no benefit by 12–24 h from onset (Fig. 2 [2]).

The Fibrinolytic Therapy Trialists (FTT) collaboration suggested that this decline in efficacy was rather linear, with little evidence of a dramatically improved benefit in the first hour (the "golden" hour), suggested by a retrospective analysis of the GISSI-1 study. However this was not seen in the prospectively stratified ISIS-2 study [2].

Simoons and colleagues [9] have revived the "golden" hour concept by adding some smaller trials (which reported data broken down by first hour effects), so producing a curvilinear rather than a linear model. It is likely that publication bias has distorted this model since several other smaller trials (not included in his model) did not report 1-h effects – presumably because they saw no particular benefit. However we are all agreed that it is important to streamline treatment protocols and emergency room procedures to eliminate the all too frequent delays in decision making and drug delivery. Simple, non-costly changes in organisation can have large effects.

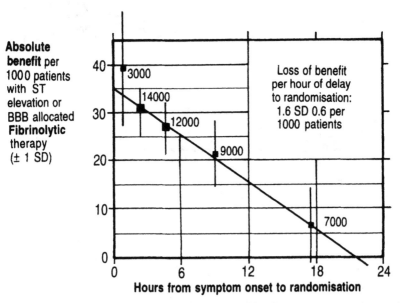

Fig. 2. Absolute reduction in 35-day morality versus delay from symptom onset to randomisation among 45,000 patients with ST elevation or BBB. (All patients in ASSET and LATE are included) For patients whose delays were recorded as 0–1, 2–3, 4–6, 7–12 and 13–24 h, absolute benefit (+A SD) is plotted against mean recorded delay time (0.98, 2.50, 4.79, 9.11 and 17.48 h, respectively.) *Area of black square* and extent to which it influences line drawn through five points is approximately proportional to number of patients it is based on (formally, area is inversely proportional to variance of absolute benefit it describes, and slope is inverse-variance-weighted least squares regression line). (With permission from [2])

Which Thrombolytic Agent?

I and my colleagues in Oxford do not believe that there are very great differences between the different thrombolytic agents [10]. GUSTO-1 appeared to show some superiority for tPA over SK or their combination, but this may be due in part to undue emphasis on one subgroup (while no similar benefit was seen, as had been expected, in the other tPA subgroup where the dosage of tPA was very similar). It is also possible that the large benefit of tPA in N. American centres in GUSTO-1 and the lesser benefit in the other non-American centres might have been due to premature stopping of SK in the N. American centres whose physicians and nurses were unused to the hypotension commonly seen with SK. This hypotension might well be beneficial since, particularly in the elderly, SK gives rise to significantly less cerebral haemorrhage than tPA. The overview of all the randomised data from large trials shows a marginal non-significant mortality advantage for tPA which in my view does not outweigh its much greater cost (Fig. 3 [10]).

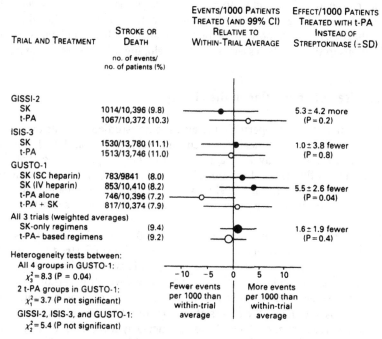

Fig. 3. Stroke or death in the three large, directly randomised comparisons (GISSI-2, ISIS-3 and GUSTO-1) of the standard streptokinase regimen with more intensive tPA-based fibrinolytic regimens. For each treatment group the number of events per 1000 patients treated (with its 99% confidence interval) is plotted, after subtraction of the overall average number of events per 1000 patients treated in that trial. *Solid circles* streptokinase-only regimens; *open symbols* tPA-based regimens. (Subtraction of the overall within-trial risk does not affect the difference between the different groups in one trial, but merely centres the results for each trial on the same vertical line.) The weighted average of the results from the three trials has weights proportional to the number of patients in those trials. *SK* Streptokinase; *SC* subcutaneous; *IV* intravenous. (With permission [10])

Some physicians prefer tPA for younger, normotensive patients, where the risk of cerebral bleeding is low; however as the absolute risk of younger patients is much lower the fiscal cost per life saved becomes very large.

tPA is of course useful for patients who have received SK for a prior MI, since there is no data on the effectiveness of SK in the presence of raised antibodies. There is no indication of excess complications when SK has been used a second time, so for those countries which cannot afford the cost of tPA for such patients my advice is to use SK on the second occasion.

Direct PTCA Is Not Superior to Thrombolysis

Although the early small trials of PTCA versus thrombolysis [3] suggested a large mortality advantage, with less stroke for PTCA, subsequent data from the much larger GUSTO-II study [11], and from many MI registries have shown no significant differences between these two modalities. Although direct PTCA is more costly and cumbersome to deliver, and although in practice it may significantly delay time to treatment, in well organised and experienced centres it certainly is an alternative to thrombolysis. It is also appropriate for the sizeable number of patients with contra-indications to thrombolytics e.g. patients developing MI after recent surgery.

Under Use of Reperfusion in the Elderly

Although many of the reperfusion trials have not studied patients over 65 years, the reality is that most clinical MI's occur in the elderly [12] and the 1 month mortality rate rises strikingly with age. The FTT analysis [2] showed that the risk reduction with the use of thrombolysis is similar to younger patients and so the absolute benefit is higher in the elderly. Despite this, and even allowing for some increase in the numbers with contra-indications there does seem to be under-usage in the elderly.

In a large US Medicare database of over 65,000 myocardial infarctions the percentage of acute MI patients receiving lytic therapy [13] fell steadily from around 30% to 5% as age increased from 55–80 [5]. This is probably driven by fear of complications, particularly cerebral haemorrhage, which is certainly somewhat higher in the elderly. However stroke also occurs in the placebo or control groups in these trials and in fact the excess of stroke caused by thrombolysis is much the same as age rises from 60–75 and over, particularly if SK is used [2]. In the FTT overview there was a highly significant 4–5-fold increase in risk from cerebral haemorrhage with tPA compared with SK in the oldest age group.

Adjunctive Treatment

ISIS-2 showed that aspirin was almost as effective as SK in reducing 35 day mortality, but that the two treatments were additive [4]. In some subgroups of patients the more effective IIb/IIIa receptor antagonists may be even more effective.

Although promising, these newer agents do seem to have greater bleeding risks and we have, at present, insufficient data to assess their safety in widespread practice. The expense of the newer agents will certainly limit their current use to higher risk patients undergoing interventions.

In routine use Heparin appears to confer a marginal mortality benefit when added to aspirin, coupled with a small increase in the risk of haemorrhagic stroke [10]. My personal advice is only to use Heparin in patients with indications due to poor LV function or arrhythmia, to prevent atrial clot formation.

Conclusion

We now have good evidence of the effectiveness of thrombolytic therapy, not only in the immediate weeks following infarction, but also, remarkably, for up to 10 years later, where the initial difference in survival appears to persist unabated.

We now know that up to 70% of Q-wave MI's occur because of thrombotic occlusion which follows the rupture of a plaque which is not causing any significant obstruction. It is this fact which is probably responsible for the remarkable effectiveness of lytic therapy.

Finally we should not neglect the 70% of patients with AMI who die outside hospital and therefore cannot receive effective reperfusion. The only way to prevent these deaths is to pursue effective secondary prevention with aspirin, statins and lifestyle advice, and population strategies to lower blood pressure and serum cholesterol as primary prevention.

References

1. Volmink JA Newton JN, Hicks NR, Sleight P, Fowler GH, Neil HAW, on behalf of the Oxford Myocardial Infarction Incidence Study Group (1998). Coronary event and case fatality rates in an English population: results of the Oxford Myocardial Infarction Incidence Study (OXMIS). Heart 80: 40–44
2. Fibrinolytic Therapy Trialists' (FTT) Collaborative Group (1994). Indications for fibrinolytic therapy in suspected acute myocardial infarction: collaborative overview of early mortality and major morbidity results from all randomised trials of more than 1000 patients. Lancet 343: 311–322
3. Grines CL, O'Neill WW. Primary angioplasty (1995). Br Heart J 73: 405–406
4. Sleight P (Chairman) ISIS-2 (Second International Study of Infarct Survival) Collaborative Group. Randomised trial of intravenous streptokinase, oral aspirin, both or neither among 17,187 cases of suspected acute myocardial infarction: ISIS-2. Lancet 1988; ii: 349–60
5. Collins R, MacMahon S, Flather M, Baigent C, Remvig L, Mortensen S, Appleby P, Godwin J, Yusuf S, Peto R. Clinical effects of anticoagulant therapy in suspected acute myocardial infarction: systematic overview of randomised trials. BMJ 1996; 313: 652–659
6. Simoons ML, de Boer MJ, van den Brand MJBM, van Miltenburg AJM, Hoorntje JCA, Heyndrickx GR, van der Wieken LR, et al. and the European Cooperative Study Group (1994). Randomized trial of a GPIIb IIIa platelet receptor blocker in refractory unstable angina. Circulation 89: 596–603
7. Hackett D, Davies G, Chierchia S, Maseri A (1987). Intermittent coronary occlusion in acute myocardial infarction. Value of combined thrombolytic and vasodilator therapy. N Engl J Med 317: 1055–1059

8. Chambless L, Keil U, Dobson A, et al. for the WHO MONICA project (1997). Population versus clinical view of case fatality from acute coronary heart disease. Results from the WHO MONICA Project 1985–1990. Circulation 96: 3849–3859

9. Boersma E, Maas AC, Deckers JW, Simoons ML (1996). Early thrombolytic treatment in acute myocardial infarction: reappraisal of the golden hour. Lancet 348: 771–775

10. Collins R, Peto R, Baigent C, Sleight P (1997). Aspirin, heparin and fibrinolytic therapy in suspected acute myocardial infarction. N Engl J Med 336: 847–860

11. The Global Use of Strategies to Open Occluded Coronary Arteries in Acute Coronary Syndromes (GUSTO IIb) Angioplasty Substudy Investigators (1997). A clinical trial comparing primary angioplasty with tissue plasminogen activator for acute myocardial infarction. N Engl J Med 336: 1621–1628

12. Gurwitz JH, Goldberg RJ, Gore JM. Coronary thrombolysis for the Elderly? (1991) JAMA 265: 1720–1723

13. Pashos CL, Normand S-LT, Garfinkle JB, Newhouse JP, Epstein AM, McNeil BJ. (1994) Trends in the use of drug therapies in patients with acute myocardial infarction: 1988–1992. JACC 23: 1023–1030

Interventional Cardiology
in the Treatment of Coronary Disease

C. Spaulding, R. Cador, S. Weber

Introduction

The first Percutaneous Transluminal Coronary Angioplasty (PTCA) in a patient was performed by Andreas Grüntzig in Zurich in September 1977 [1]. PTCA was initially limited to the treatment of discrete stenosis in proximal segments of a coronary artery. Improvements in equipment and technique have increased the success rate and have lead to its use in patients with complex stenosis or high-risk clinical situations such as unstable angina, acute myocardial infarction [2, 3], or cardiac arrest [4]. PTCA is currently the most widely used coronary revascularization technique and over 1,000,000 procedures were performed worldwide in 1996 [5].

Peformance of the Procedure

Successful PTCA requires a skilled operator and high-resolution fluoroscopic equipment. Vascular access is usually obtained through the femoral artery where a sheath is introduced with the use of local anesthesia. A 6–9 French guide catheter (2–3 mm in diameter) is advanced through the sheath to the ostium of the coronary artery to be dilated (Fig. 1). Once the guiding catheter is positioned in the coronary ostium, angiography of the diseased artery is performed to visu-

Fig. 1. Femoral approach. The guiding catheter is introduced through a femoral arterial sheath and advanced to the ostium of the diseased coronary artery

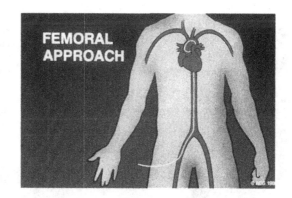

alize the stenosis and the arterial segments proximal and distal to it. A flexible guide wire is advanced through the guiding catheter, navigated across the stenosis by rotating and advancing its angulated tip and positioned in the distal arterial segment. With the guide wire across the stenosis, the deflated balloon catheter is advanced over the wire and positioned at the stenosis. The positions of the guide wire and balloon catheter are confirmed periodically by visualization of the artery by injecting contrast medium through the guiding catheter. Once positioned, the balloon is usually inflated for 1–2 min at 3–12 atm pressure with a mixture of saline and contrast medium so that the inflation can be visualized.

Many patients have angina, electrocardiographic evidence of ischemia, or both during balloon inflation since the coronary artery is temporarily occluded. Most often, a stent is implanted after balloon angioplasty. Balloon expandable stents are most commonly used. The stent is crimped on a balloon, the device is positioned on the stenosis and the stent implanted in the coronary artery wall by a short balloon inflation (Fig. 2). The balloon catheter is then pulled out and the result is evaluated by injecting contrast medium. If the result is satisfactory, the guide wire is removed. If the dilatation is not adequate, the guide wire remains in place and the balloon catheter can be replaced by a larger one or another stent may be implanted (Fig. 2). At the end of the procedure, a final angiogram is obtained to confirm that the result is satisfactory and that the other segments of the artery, including branches, have not been compromised.

Medications, Pre- and Post-procedure Mamangement

Low-dose aspirin has been shown to reduce the incidence of acute occlusion after PTCA and is considered essential therapy prior to non-emergent interventions [6]. A dose of 160–325 mg of aspirin is therefore given before and after PTCA For patients allergic to aspirin, ticlopidine is a reasonable alternative but should be initiated 5 days before PTCA to obtain the maximal antiplatelet effect. Heparin (typically 7500–10 000 units) is administered intravenously during the procedure to decrease the incidence of coronary artery thrombosis [7] but is usually not

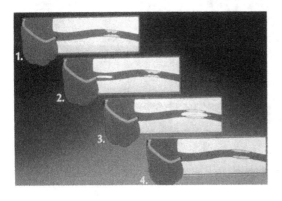

Fig. 2. PTCA procedure. 1 The guiding catheter is positioned in the ostium of the coronary artery. 2 The guide wire is advanced across the stenosis. 3 The balloon is slid forward on the guide wire, positioned on the stenosis and inflated. 4 After one or more inflations, the guide wire and balloon catheters are removed and a final angiogram is performed

continued after the procedure. Intracoronary nitrates are given at the beginning and during the procedure to prevent vasospasm.

After PTCA, the femoral arterial sheath is removed 4–8 h after the procedure, once the anticoagulant effect of the heparin dissipates. The patient remains in bed for 8–24 h. If the procedure has been uncomplicated, the patient is often discharged the day after the removal of the sheath. Medications prescribed at the time of the discharge depend on the underlying condition. Most often, post-PTCA regimen includes low-dose aspirin, a beta-blocker or a calcium antagonist, and long-lasting nitrates. If a stent has been implanted, a combination of low-dose aspirin (80–325 mg per day) and ticlopidine (500 mg per day) significantly reduces the rate of stent-associated thrombosis [8] and is prescribed for 4 weeks after the procedure.

Although the femoral artery remains the most widely used approach for diagnostic and therapeutic procedures, the radial artery is used increasingly to reduce the local complication rate and increase the patient's comfort. The sheath is pulled out immediately after the procedure and hemostasis is obtained by applying a pressure dressing for several hours [9]. Immediate ambulation is feasible and hospital discharge is possible in selected cases [10].

Efficacy of the Procedure

With modern equipment, PTCA of a nonoccluded coronary artery is successful in more than 95% of patients [11]. In the remaining patients, PTCA is unsuccessful because the stenosis cannot be crossed with either the guide wire or the balloon catheter or the stenosis is not adequately dilated despite the use of a balloon of appropriate size and stents. In around 3–5% cases the vessel abruptly occludes (abrupt closure) during or immediately after the procedure. Reopening of the artery is attempted with repeat balloon inflations. If this fails, a coronary stent is implanted. Stenting for abrupt closure (bailout stenting) has virtually eliminated the need for urgent coronary bypass surgery after failed PTCA. Coronary angioplasty has a lower success rate with stenosis that are long, angulated, calcified, or associated with intraluminal thrombus [12, 13]. PTCA also has a lower initial success rate (50–70%) in patients with chronically occluded arteries than in those with narrowed arteries, since it may be difficult to manipulate the guide wire through a chronically occluded region [14, 15]. In patients with recurrent angina after bypass surgery, the PTCA success rate of properly selected stenosis of saphenous and arterial bypass grafts is close to that of native arteries, but the incidence of late events (myocardial infarction, repeat PTCA or surgery) is higher [16, 17].

Mechanisms of Arterial Dilatation

The mechanisms by which PTCA increases the size of the arterial lumen have been studied in animals and cadavers [18, 19, 20, 21]. Balloon-induced barotrauma causes endothelial denudation, cracking and disruption of the atherosclerotic plaque, and stretching or tearing of the media and adventitia (Fig. 3). These brutal and profound changes account for the post-PTCA angiographic features of intraluminal haziness, intimal flap or dissection. Intracoronary ultrasound imaging, which provides a cross-sectional view of the artery within the lumen, detects dissection of the arterial wall – at times extensive – in 50–80% of patients who have undergone successful PTCA [22, 23]. These morphological alterations open up new pathways for blood flow, leading to an increased luminal size. Balloon inflation may be deleterious, however, causing plaque hemorrhage, extensive dissection resulting in luminal compromise, platelet deposition or thrombus formation.

In the weeks after successful PTCA, favorable remodeling of the disrupted plaque and endothelialization at the sites of intimal injury result in an increased luminal size. Angiographic studies indicate that intimal disruption usually resolves within 1 month after successful PTCA [24].

Restenosis

In patients who have undergone successful PTCA, recurrence of the stenosis, or restenosis, is the main limitation to long-term, event-free survival. Several definitions of restenosis have been suggested, but it is most commonly defined as more than a 50% narrowing of the diameter of the lumen at the site of a previously successful PTCA. Restenosis occurs in about one third of patients in whom a coronary artery stenosis has been dilated by balloon alone [25–27]. Restenosis typically occurs one to 6 months after PTCA [25].

The process of restenosis is multifactorial. Injury of the vessel initiates release of thrombogenic, vasoactive and mitogenic factors [28]. Endothelial and deep-vessel injury leads to platelet aggregation, thrombus formation, inflammation and activation of macrophages and smooth-muscle cells. These events induce the production and release of growth factors and cytokines, which in turn may promote their own synthesis, and release from target cells [29]. A self-perpetuating process is initiates, which results in the migration of smooth-muscle cells from their usual location in the arterial media to the intima, where they change to a synthetic phenotype, produce extracellular matrix, and proliferate, thereby resulting in a stenosis within the vessel lumen. Intimal thickening accounts for about 30% of the loss in lumen diameter 6 months after coronary interventions. In addition, arterial remodeling occurs in the weeks after PTCA and can be measured using serial intravascular ultrasound imaging after PTCA to measure the reduction in the cross-sectional area of the vessel [30, 31].

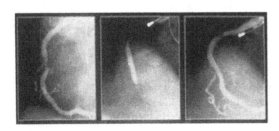

Fig. 3. PTCA of a right coronary artery. *Right* Stenosis on the mid-segment of the right coronary artery; *middle* balloon inflation; *left* final result

More than 70 trials enrolling more than 15,000 patients have evaluated various drugs to block intimal proliferation after PTCA [32]. Only one trial, using probucol, has shown beneficial results [33]. However probucol must be administered 1 month before the procedure. In contrast, coronary stenting significantly reduces the incidence of restenosis because it produces large lumens and staves off pathological remodeling [34, 35].

New Devices

Coronary Stenting

Coronary stents are fenestrated stainless-steel tubes that can be expanded by a balloon and provide scaffold within coronary arteries (Fig. 3). Coronary stenting has virtually eliminated the immediate need for urgent bypass for abrupt vessel closure during PTCA by sealing intimal flaps and dissections against the vessel wall [36, 37, 38]. Stents also reduce the likelihood of restenosis. Several multicenter randomized trials showed that the incidence of restenosis was 25–50% lower after coronary stenting than after PTCA for de novo lesions in large native lesions measuring 3.0 mm or more in diameter [34, 35].

Subacute thrombotic occlusion of coronary stents occurs in about 1% of patients. In contrast to complete vessel closure, which most often occurs during or immediately after the procedure, stent occlusion happens within 2–14 days after stent implantation [34, 35, 39]. Initial efforts to prevent stent thrombosis included an intensive anticoagulation regimen with high dose heparin during stent implantation and warfarin after the procedure which resulted in high bleeding complication rates [34, 35]. Alternative methods were then investigated. Inhibition of platelet activation by an association of ticlopidine and aspirin was shown to be effective in preventing subacute stent thrombosis with a low bleeding complication rate in several French registries [40, 41] and in a German randomized trial [8] (Table 1). The current post-stenting regimen associates ticlopidine 500 mg per day and aspirin, 80–325 mg per day. Ticlopidine is discontinued after 4 weeks. Neutropenia occurs in around 1% of cases and most often resolves after discontinuation of ticlopidine [8, 40, 41]. Intracoronary ultrasound imaging performed during stent implantation allows adequate stent expansion, significantly reduces the rate of subacute stent occlusion and has been suggested as an alternative to anticoagulation and inhibition of platelet activation [42]. However, routine use of intracoronary ultrasound is time-consuming and increases the procedure costs.

The use of coronary stents is rising dramatically and the number of stent-implantation procedures is currently exceeding that of conventional balloon angioplasty procedures in most European countries. More than 20 new stent designs are currently available or under investigation (Figs. 4–6).

Table 1. Randomized comparison of antiplatelet therapy with aspirin and ticlopidine and anti-coagulant therapy: end points and events (from [8])

Event	Antiplatelet therapy (%)	Anticoagulant therapy (%)	p
Primary cardiac endpoint	1.6	6.2	0.01
Death	0.4	0.8	1.0
Myocardial infarction	0.8	4.2	0.02
Reintervention	1.2	5.4	0.01
Primary noncardiac endpoint	1.2	12.3	<0.001
Death	0	0	–
Cerebrovascular accident	0.4	0	1.0
Hemorrhagic event	0	6.5	<0.001
Peripheral vascular event	0.8	6.2	0.001
Combined clinical endpoint	2.7	5.4	<0.001
Occlusion of stented vessel	0.8	0.4	0.004

Directional Atherectomy, Laser Angioplasty, and Rotational Atherectomy

Directional atherectomy extracts atherosclerotic tissue from the coronary artery with a cutting blade spinning at 5000 rpm in the tip of the atherectomy device [43]. During laser angioplasty, light emitted from optical fibers at the catheter tip vaporizes atheromatous tissue [44]. Rotational atherectomy uses a diamond-studded burr spinning at about 180,000 rpm to excavate calcified or fibrotic plaque [45]. In several randomized trials, these new devices have not reduced the rates late clinical events after coronary angioplasty [46, 47, 48].

Catheter-Based Radiotherapy

In animal models of coronary restenosis, intracoronary radiotherapy has been shown to reduce intimal hyperplasia. In a preliminary study on patients with previous coronary restenosis, coronary stenting followed by catheter-based intra-coronary radiotherapy substantially reduced the rate of subsequent restenosis [49]. Further randomized trials are under way.

Use of Antithrombotic Therapies During Coronary Angioplasty

Although the mainstay of anticoagulation therapy during PTCA remains the combination of aspirin and heparin during the procedure, several new antithrombotic therapies for PTCA have been tested.

Fig. 4. Coronary stenting with a
Palmaz-Schatz coronary stent

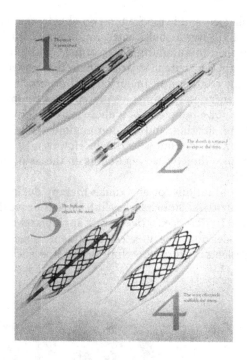

Fig. 5. Mechanisms of arterial
dilatation. Coronary artery
dissection created by a single
balloon inflation

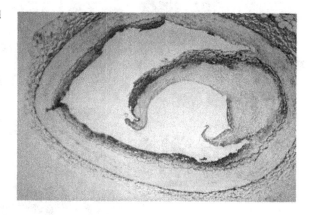

Multicenter studies evaluated direct thrombin inhibitors in patients undergoing PTCA for unstable angina and found that these agents were only marginally better than heparin in preventing ischemic complications [50, 51]. The failure of thrombin inhibitors is now attributed to the multiplicity of pathways for
platelet activation and the inability of these agents, in contrast to heparin, to
block the generation of heparin. Whereas there are multiple pathways for
platelet activation, a single receptor mediates the process of platelet aggregation. The platelet glycoprotein IIb/IIIa receptor binds fibrinogen to cross-link

platelets and is blocked irreversibly by the monoclonal antibody abciximab or c7E3. Several multicenter randomized studies have compared heparin and aspirin to an additional treatment with abciximab in patients with unstable angina or acute myocardial infarction undergoing PTCA and showed a significant reduction in major clinical events at 1 month in patients [52–57]. In a recent trial, stenting plus placebo was compared to stenting plus abciximab, or balloon angioplasty plus abciximab. Abciximab significantly increased the safety of stenting, and balloon angioplasty with abciximab was even safer than stenting without abciximab. However, complication rates were high in all groups thereby casting doubts on the definition of major complications in this trial [58].

Indications for abciximab therapy during coronary angioplasty are clearly evolving. Although large clinical trials prove that blockade of platelet glycoprotein IIb/IIIa is effective during angioplasty optimal patient selection remains to be defined. The greatest treatment benefit of abciximab appears to be in patients with severe clinical patterns such as unstable angina refractory to

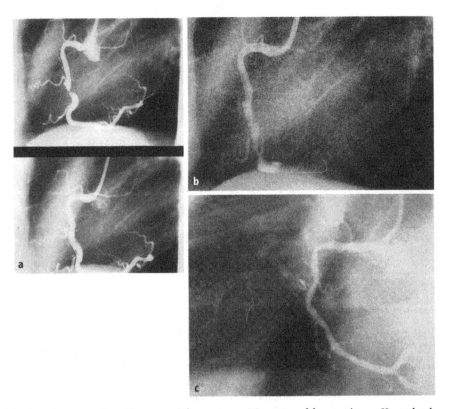

Fig. 6a–c. Coronary dissection on a right coronary artery treated by stenting. **a** *Upper level* before angioplasty; *lower level* coronary dissection after one balloon inflation. **b** Coronary occlusion occurring 5 min after the balloon inflation. **c** Final result after stent implantation

medical treatment and acute myocardial infarction. In all cases, abciximab must be started at the beginning of the procedure and not once complications arise.

Clinical Applications

Choosing among medical therapy, angioplasty and surgical treatments remains a difficult decision in the care of individual patients with coronary artery disease. Nonetheless, the results of several clinical trials allow general guidelines to be developed.

PTCA Versus Medical Therapy

PTCA has been compared with medical therapy for stable angina in several studies. In the Angioplasty Compared with Medicine study, patients with stable angina and single-vessel coronary disease were randomly assigned to treatment with PTCA or medical therapy [59, 60]. In the Medicine, Angioplasty or Surgery study, patients with stable angina and a stenosis of the proximal left anterior descending artery were randomly assigned to medical therapy, PTCA, or bypass surgery with the left internal thoracic artery [61]. The Randomized Intervention Treatment of Angina (RITA-2) trial compared the long-term effects of PTCA and medical care in patients with coronary artery disease considered suitable for either treatment [62]. The Asymptomatic Cardiac Ischemia Pilot (ACIP) study randomized patients to three treatment strategies: angina-guided drug therapy, angina plus ischemia-guided drug therapy or revascularization by angioplasty or bypass surgery [63]. These studies suggested that PTCA provides more complete relief of angina than medical therapy.

The TIMI IIIB study addressed the benefit of PTCA for patients with unstable angina or non-Q-wave myocardial infarction. An aggressive strategy of early cardiac catheterization with angioplasty was compared with a conservative strategy of medical therapy for patients presenting with ischemic pain at rest. Although major complications occurred with similar frequencies in patients assigned to the two groups, more post-discharge procedures and hospitalizations were required by the patients assigned to the conservative strategy, suggesting that PTCA provides more rapid and complete relief of angina without increasing the risk of major complications [64, 65].

Several studies have evaluated PTCA in patients with acute myocardial infarction [66, 67, 68] and showed that PTCA, performed without prior thrombolytic therapy (primary PTCA) by experienced teams results in a lower risk of death or reinfarction than thrombolytic therapy (Table 2). Stenting during primary angioplasty for acute myocardial infarction further reduces the occurrence of adverse events at 1 month [69, 70, 71]. In cardiac arrest, a strategy of immediate coronary angiography followed if necessary by angioplasty may increase survival [4]. Finally, PTCA performed after failed thrombolytic therapy reduces adverse cardiac events and improves left ventricular function at 1 month [72, 73].

Thus, the results of clinical trials comparing PTCA with medical therapy suggest that the benefit of angioplasty depends on the severity and acuity of the clinical presentation. A gradient of risk extends across the spectrum of patients with coronary artery disease. At one end of the spectrum, patients with stable angina and one or two-vessel disease treated medically are at low risk of nonfatal myocardial infarction. PTCA reduces angina more effectively with a low risk of complications, but does not lower the risk of death, myocardial infarction, or future revascularization procedures. In daily practice initial revascularization by PTCA is therefore proposed in this setting if the amount of myocardium at risk is high and if the lesions seem at low risk for procedure related complications. At the other end of the spectrum, patients with acute myocardial infarction have a risk of major complications and death that can be drastically reduced by primary PTCA. In the middle of the spectrum, patients with unstable angina have an intermediate risk of major ischemic complications. In this setting, PTCA provides symptomatic relief and stabilizes the course of unstable angina.

PTCA Versus Bypass Surgery

Several studies have compared PTCA with bypass surgery for patients with multi-vessel coronary artery disease. Despite the use of different protocols, the studies have yielded consistent results [74–79]. Major complications, such as death or myocardial infarction, occur with similar frequencies one to 5 years after angioplasty or bypass surgery (Table 3). However, there is an increased need for repeat revascularization procedures in patients who are randomized to PTCA. Furthermore in the BARI study, diabetic patients had higher rates of survival 5 years after treatment with bypass surgery [75]. New randomized trials comparing angioplasty with bypass surgery are now been performed with the use of stents.

In daily practice, most patients with multi-vessel disease have diffuse lesions or chronic occlusions that are not amendable to PTCA. Bypass surgery therefore remains the preferred therapeutic option in this subset of patients such as those

Table 2. Randomized comparison of primary angioplasty and thrombolytic therapy for acute myocardial infarction: the PAMI study (*low risk* patients withoug high-risk factors, *low risk* patients older than 70, with an anterior infarction, or a heart rate of more than 100 bpm on admission; from [2])

Event	PTCA group (%)	t-PA group (%)	p
Reinfarction	2.6	6.5	0.06
Death	2.6	6.5	0.06
Low risk	3	2	0.69
High risk	2	11	0.001
Nonfatal reinfarction or death	5.1	12	0.02

Table 3. Comparison of surgical therapy and coronary angioplasty: Five-year results of the BARI study (*CABG* coronary artery bypass surgery, *PTCA* percutaneous transluminal coronary angioplasty, *MI* myocardial infarction; from [75])

Endpoint	CABG (%)	PTCA (%)
Death	10.7	13.7
Death or MI	19.6	21.3
Repeated CABG	0.7	20.5*
Repeated CABG or PTCA	8.0	54.0*

*$P<0.05$

with left main and triple-vessel coronary artery disease with critical obstruction of the proximal left anterior descending artery and/or left ventricular dysfunction. Non-diabetic patients with multi-vessel coronary disease that are good candidates for either PTCA or bypass surgery can be reassured that both revascularization approaches are followed by equivalent rates of major complications. However, the invasive nature of bypass surgery must be weighed against the likelihood of repeated procedures after PTCA. Whether stenting will reduce the rate of reintervention after angioplasty in patients with multivessel disease remains to be proven by on-going trials

Conclusion

In the past decade, PTCA has emerged as the most widely used method of coronary revascularization. It immediately suppresses anginal symptoms in patients with stable and unstable angina and significantly reduces mortality and morbidity rates in patients with acute myocardial infarction. Coronary stenting has revolutionized the practice of interventional cardiology by partially overcoming the limitations of coronary angioplasty, such as abrupt vessel closure and restenosis. Ongoing studies of optimal antithrombotic therapies may improve the success rate of coronary stent implantation and further reduce the risk of major complications.

With this enhanced technologic prowess, reasoned judgement in the management of patients remains necessary. Angioplasty should be viewed as a part of a comprehensive strategy against coronary artery disease with through application of appropriate therapies at the appropriate times, be they medical, interventional or surgical. In the final analysis, only patient outcomes determine the success of our efforts.

References

1. Gruntzig A (1978) Transluminal dilatation of coronary-artery stenosis. Lancet 1:263
2. Grines CL, Browne KF, Marco J, et al. (1993) Comparison of immediate angioplasty with thrombolytic therapy for acute myocardial infarction. N Engl J Med 328:673–9

3. Zijlstra F, de Boer MJ, Hoomtje JCA, Reiffers S, et al. (1993) A comparaison of immediate coronary angioplasty with intravenous streptokinase in acute myocardial infarction. N Engl J Med 328:680–4
4. Spaulding CM, Joly LM, Rosenberg A, et al. (1997) Immediate coronary angiography in survivors of out-of-hospital cardiac arrest. N Engl J Med 336:1629–33
5. Bittl JA (1996) Advances in coronary angioplasty. N Engl J Med 335:1290–1302
6. Barnathan ES, Schwartz JS, Taylor L, et al. (1987) Aspirin and dipyridamole in the prevention of acute coronary thrombosis complicating coronary angioplasty. Circulation 76:125–34
7. McGarry TF Jr, Gottlieb RS, Morganroth J, et al. (1992) The relationship of anticoagulation level and complications after successful percutaneous transluminal coronary angioplasty. Am Heart J 123:1445–51
8. Schomig A, Neumann FJ, Kastrati A, et al. (1996) Randomized comparison of antiplatelet and anticoagulant therapy after the placement of coronary-artery stents. N Engl J Med 334:1084–9
9. Spaulding C, Lefèvre T, Funck F, et al. (1996) Left Radial Approach for Coronary Angiography: Results of a Prospective Trial. Cath Cardiovasc Diagn 39:365–70
10. Kiemeneij F, Laarman GJ, Slagboom T, van der Wieken R (1997) Outpatient coronary stent implantation. J Am Coll Cardiol 29:323–7
11. Ellis SG (1990) Elective coronary angioplasty: technique and complications. In: Topol EJ, ed. Textbook of interventional cardiology. Philadelphia: W.B. Saunders, pp 200–1
12. Ellis SG, Roubin GS, King SP III, et al. (1988) In-hospital mortality after acute closure after coronary angioplasty: Analysis of risk factors from 8,207 procedures. J Am Coll Cardiol 11:211–216
13. Kimmel SE, Berlin JA, Strom BL, Laskey WK (1995) Development and validation of a simplified predictive index for major complications in contemporary percutaneous transluminal coronary angioplasty practice. J Am Coll Cardiol 26:931–38
14. Bell MR, Berger PB, Bresnahan JF, Reeder GS, Bailey KR, Holmes DR Jr (1992) Initial and long-term outcome of 354 patients after coronary balloon angioplasty of total coronary artery occlusions. Circulation 85:1003–11.
15. Ivanhoe RJ, Weintraub WS, Douglas JS Jr, et al. (1992) Percutaneous transluminal coronary angioplasty of chronic total occlusions: primary success, restenosis, and long-term clinical follow-up. Circulation 85:106–15.
16. de Feyter PJ, van Suylen R-J, de Jaegere PPT, Topol EJ, Serruys PW (1993) Balloon angioplasty for the treatment of lesions in saphenous vein bypass grafts. J Am Coll Cardiol 21:1539–49
17. Savage MP, Douglas JS Jr, Fischman DL, et al. (1997) Stent placement compared with balloon angioplasty for obstructed coronary bypass grafts. N Engl J Med 337:740–7
18. Faxon DP, Weber VJ, Haudenschild C, Gottsman SB, McGovern WA, Ryan TJ (1982) Acute effects of transluminal angioplasty in three experimental models of atherosclerosis. Arteriosclerosis 2:125–33
19. Steele PM, Chesebro JH, Stanson AW, et al. (1985) Balloon angioplasty: natural history of the pathophysiological response to injury in a pig model. Circ Res 57:105–12
20. Farb A, Virmani R, Atkinson JB, Kolodgie FD (1990) Plaque morphology and pathologic changes in arteries from patients dying after coronary balloon angioplasty. J Am Coll Cardiol16:1421–9
21. Soward AL, Essed CE, Serruys PW (1985) Coronary arterial findings after accidental death immediately after successful percutaneous transluminal coronary angioplasty. Am J Cardiol 56:794–5
22. Tenaglia AN, Buller CE, Kisslo KB, Stack RS, Davidson CJ (1982) Mechanisms of balloon angioplasty and directional coronary atherectomy as assessed by intracoronary ultrasound. J Am Coll Cardiol 20:685–91
23. Potkin BN, Keren G, Mintz GS, et al. (1992) Arterial responses to balloon coronary angioplasty: an intravascular ultrasound study. J Am Coll Cardiol 20:942–51
24. Waller BF (1983) Early and late morphologic changes in human coronary arteries after percutaneous transluminal coronary angioplasty. Clin Cardiol 6:363–72

25. Nobuyoshi M, Kimura T, Nosaka H, et al. (1988) Restenosis after successful percutaneous transluminal coronary angioplasty: serial angiographic follow-up of 229 patients. J Am Coll Cardiol 12:616–23

26. MERCATOR Study Group (1992) Does the new angiotensin converting enzyme inhibitor cilazapril prevent restenosis after percutaneous transluminal coronary angioplasty? Results of the MERCATOR study: a multicenter, randomized, double-blind placebo-controlled trial. Circulation 86:100–10

27. Hirshfeld JW Jr, Schwartz JS, Jugo R, et al. (1991) Restenosis after coronary angioplasty: a multivariate statistical model to relate lesion and procedure variables to restenosis. J Am Coll Cardiol 18:647–56

28. Lange RA, Willard JE, Hillis LD (1993) Restenosis: the Achilles heel of coronary angioplasty. Am J Med Sci 306:265–75

29. Libby P, Schwartz D, Brogi E, Tanaka H, Clinton SK (1992) A cascade model for restenosis: a special case of atherosclerosis progression. Circulation 86:Suppl III:III-47-III-52

30. Mintz GS, Popma JJ, Pichard AD, et al. (1996) Intravascular ultrasound predictors of restenosis after percutaneous transcatheter coronary revascularization. J Am Coll Cardiol 27:1678–87

31. Mintz GS, Popma JJ, Pichard AD, et al. (1996) Arterial remodeling after coronary angioplasty: a serial intravascular ultrasound study. Circulation 94:35–43

32. Currier JW, Faxon DP (1995) Restenosis after percutaneous transluminal coronary angioplasty: have we been aiming at the wrong target? J Am Coll Cardiol 25:516–20

33. Tardif JC, Cote G, Lesperance J, et al. (1997) Probucol and multivitamins in the prevention of restenosis after coronary angioplasty. N Engl J Med 337:365–72

34. Serruys PW, de Jaegere P, Kiemeneij F, et al. (1994) A comparison of balloon-expandable-stent implantation with balloon angioplasty in patients with coronary artery disease. N Engl J Med 331:489–95

35. Fischman DL, Leon MB, Baim DS, et al. (1994) A randomized comparison of coronary-stent placement and balloon angioplasty in the treatment of coronary artery disease. N Engl J Med 331:496–501

36. de Muinck ED, den Heijer P, van Dijk RB, et al. (1994) Autoperfusion balloon versus stent for acute or threatened closure during percutaneous transluminal coronary angioplasty. Am J Cardiol 74:1002–5

37. Lincoff AM, Topol EJ, Chapekis AT, et al. (1993) Intracoronary stenting compared with conventional therapy for abrupt vessel closure complicating coronary angioplasty: a matched case-control study. J Am Coll Cardiol 21:866–75

38. Roubin GS, Cannon AD, Agrawal SK, et al. (1992) Intracoronary stenting for acute and threatened closure complicating percutaneous transluminal coronary angioplasty. Circulation 85:916–27

39. Mak K-H, Belli G, Ellis SG, Moliterno DJ (1996) Subacute stent thrombosis: evolving issues and current concepts. J Am Coll Cardiol 27:494–503

40. Karillon GJ, Morice MC, Benveniste E, et al. (1996) Intracoronary stent implantation without ultrasound guidance and with replacement of conventional anticoagulation by antiplatelet therapy. 30-day clinical outcome of the French Multicenter Registry. Circulation 94:1519–27

41. Morice MC, Zeymour G, Benveniste E, et al. (1995) Intracoronary stenting without coumadin: one month results of a French multicenter study. Cathet Cardiovasc Diagn 35:1–7

42. Colombo A, Hall P, Nakamura S, et al. (1995) Intracoronary stenting without anticoagulation accomplished with intravascular ultrasound guidance. Circulation 91:1676–88

43. Bittl JA (1993) Directional coronary atherectomy versus balloon angioplasty. N Engl J Med 329:273–4

44. Mintz GS, Kovach JA, Javier SP, et al. (1995) Mechanisms of lumen enlargement after excimer laser coronary angioplasty: an intravascular ultrasound study. Circulation 92:3408–14

45. Safian RD, Niazi KA, Strzelecki M, et al. (1993) Detailed angiographic analysis of high-speed mechanical rotational atherectomy in human coronary arteries. Circulation 88:961–8

46. Baim DS, Cutlip DE, Sharma SK, et al. (1998) Final results of the Balloon vs Optimal Atherectomy Trial. Circulation 97:322–31

47. Simonton CA, Leon MB, Baim DS, et al. (1998) Optimal directional coronary atherectomy: final results of the Optimal Atherectomy Restenosis Study (OARS). Circulation 97:332–9

48. Reifart N, Vandormael M, Krajcar M, et al. (1997) Randomized comparison of angioplasty of complex coronary lesions at a single center: Eximer Laser, Rotational Atherectomy, and Balloon Angioplasty Comparison (ERBAC) study. Circulation 96:91–8

49. Terstein PS, Masullo V, Jani S, et al. (1997) Catheter-based radiotherapy to inhibit restenosis after coronary stenting. N Engl J Med 336:1697–703

50. Serruys PW, Herrman J PR, Simon R, et al. (1995) A comparison of hirudin with heparin in the prevention of coronary restenosis after coronary angioplasty. N Engl J Med 333: 757–63

51. Bittl JA, Strony J, Brinker JA, et al. (1995) Treatment with bivalirudin (Hirulog) as compared with heparin during coronary angioplasty for unstable or postinfarction angina. N Engl J Med 333:764–9

52. The EPIC Investigators (1994) Use of a monoclonal antibody directed against the platelet glycoprotein IIb/IIIa receptor in high-risk coronary angioplasty. N Engl J Med 330:956–61

53. Topol EJ, Califf RM, Weisman HF, et al. (1994) Randomized trial of coronary intervention with antibody against platelet IIb/IIIa integrin for reduction of clinical restenosis: results at six months. Lancet 343:881–6

54. The EPILOG Investigators (1997) Platelet glycoprotein IIb/IIIa receptor blockade and low-dose heparin during percutaneous coronary revascularization. N Engl J Med 336:1689–96

55. The IMPACT II Investigators (1997) Randomized placebo-controlled trial of the effect of eptifibatide on complications of percutaneous coronary intervention. Lancet 349:1422–8

56. The RESTORE Investigators (1997) Effects of platelet glycoprotein IIb/IIIa blockade with tirofiban on adverse cardiac events in patients with unstable angina of acute myocardial infarction undergoing coronary angioplasty. Circulation 96:1445–53

57. The CAPTURE Investigators (1997) Randomized placebo-controlled trial of abciximab before and during intervention in refractors unstable angina: the CAPTURE study. Lancet 349:1429–35

58. The EPISTENT Investigators (1998) Randomized placebo-controlled and balloon-angioplasty-controlled trial to assess safety of coronary stenting with the use of platelet glycoprotein IIb/IIIa blockade. Lancet 352:87–92

59. Parisi AF, Folland ED, Hartigan PA (1992) A comparison of angioplasty with medical therapy in the treatment of single-vessel coronary artery disease. N Engl J Med 326:10–16

60. Veterans Affairs ACME Investigators (1997) Percutaneous transluminal coronary angioplasty versus medical therapy for stable angina pectoris: outcomes for patients with double-vessel versus single-vessel coronary artery disease in a Veterans Affairs cooperative randomized trial. J Am Coll Cardiol 7:1505–11

61. Hueb WA, Belloti G, de Oliveira SA, et al. (1995) The Medicine, Angioplasty, or Surgery Study (MASS): a prospective, randomized trial of medical therapy, balloon angioplasty or bypass surgery for single proximal left anterior descending artery stenosis. J Am Coll Cardiol 26:1600–5

62. RITA-2 Trial Participants (1997) Coronary angioplasty versus medical therapy for angina: The second Randomized Interventional Treatment of Angina (RITA-2) trial. Lancet 350:461–8

63. Davies RF, Goldberg AD, Forman S, et al. (1997) Asymptomatic Cardiac Ischemia Pilot (ACIP) study two-year follow-up: outcomes of patients randomized to initial strategies of medical therapy versus revascularization. Circulation 95: 2037–43

64. The TIMI IIIB Investigators (1994) Effects of tissue plasminogen activator and a comparison of early invasive and conservative strategies in unstable angina and non-Q-wave myocardial infarction. Circulation 89:1545–56

65. Andreson HV, Cannon CP, Stone PH, et al. (1995) One-year results of the Thrombolysis in Myocardial Infarction (TIMI) IIB clinical trial: a randomized comparison of tissue-type plasminogen activator versus placebo and early invasive versus early conservative strategies in unstable angina and non-Q-wave myocardial infarction. J Am Coll Cardiol 91:476–85

66. Grines CL, Browne KF, Marco J, et al. (1993) A comparison of immediate angioplasty with thrombolytic therapy for acute myocardial infarction. The Primary Angioplasty in Myocardial Infarction Study Group. N Engl J Med 328:673–9
67. Zijlstra F, De Boer MJ, Hoorntje JC, et al. (1993) A comparison of immediate coronary angioplasty with intravenous streptokinase in acute myocardial infarction. N Engl J Med 328:680–4
68. The GUSTO IIb angioplasty substudy investigators (1997) A clinical trial comparing primary coronary angioplasty with tissue plasminogen activator for acute myocardial infarction. N Engl J Med 336:1621–8
69. Garcia-Cantu E, Spaulding C, Corcos T et al. Stent implantation in acute myocardial infarction. Am J Cardiol 1996; 77: 451–4.
70. Spaulding C, Cador R, Benhamda K et al. (1997) One week and six-month angiographic controls of stent implantation for occlusive and non-occlusive dissection occurring during primary balloon angioplasty for acute myocardial infarction. Am J Cardiol 79: 1592–1595
71. Rodriguez A, Bernardi V, Fernandez M, et al. (1998) In-hospital and late results of coronary stents versus conventional balloon angioplasty in acute myocardial infarction (GRAMI trial). Gianturco-Roubin in Acute Myocardial Infarction. Am J Cardiol 81:1286–91
72. The CORAMI study group (1994) Outcome of attempted rescue angioplasty after failed thrombolysis for acute myocardial infarction. Am J Cardiol 74:172–4
73. Ellis SG, Ribero Da Silva E, Heyndrickx G, et al. (1994) Randomized comparison of rescue angioplasty with conservative management of patients with early failure of thrombolysis for acute myocardial infarction. Circulation 90:2280–4
74. King SB III, Lembo NJ, Weintraub WS, et al. (1994) A randomized trial comparing coronary angioplasty with coronary bypass surgery. N Engl J Med 331:1044–50
75. The Bypass Angioplasty Revascularization Investigation (BARI) Investigators (1996) Comparison of coronary bypass surgery with angioplasty in patients with multivessel disease. N Engl J Med 335:217–25
76. CABRI trial participants (1995) Coronary Angioplasty vs. Bypass Revascularization Investigation (CABRI) results during the first year. Lancet 346:1179–83
77. RITA Trial Participants (1993) Coronary angioplasty versus coronary artery bypass surgery: The Randomized Intervention Treatment of Angina (RITA) trial. Lancet 341:573–80
78. Hamm CW, Reimers J, Ischinger T, et al. (1994) A randomized study of coronary angioplasty compared with bypass surgery in patients with symptomatic multivessel coronary artery disease. N Engl J Med 334:1037–43
79. Rodriguez A, Bouillon F, Perz-Balino N, et al. (1993) Argentine randomized trial of percutaneous transluminal coronary angioplasty versus coronary artery bypass surgery in multivessel disease (ERACI): in-hospital results and 1-year follow-up. J Am Coll Cardiol 33:1060–7

Enhancement of Coronary Blood Flow as Myocardial Salvage Therapy

D. Karila-Cohen

Introduction

The early and late prognosis of acute myocardial infarction are mainly related to the final infarct size, which is the total amount of left ventricular myocardial necrosis. The potentially maximal infarct size is the area at risk, which is the amount of jeopardized myocardium during coronary artery occlusion. The area of necrosis spreads from the center of the area at risk toward its periphery. The aim of reperfusion therapy is to stop the progression of necrosis by restoring coronary blood flow as early as possible. This limitation of infarct size represents myocardial salvage, and is associated with improved prognosis. The aim of this chapter is to describe the implications of improving coronary blood flow during the acute phase of myocardial infarction on myocardial salvage, and thus on global prognosis.

The Problem

Epicardial Coronary Patency

In clinical practice, "coronary recanalization" is considered as the goal of reperfusion therapy, and as the best and easier way to assess semi-quantitatively "coronary blood flow". Nevertheless, this introduces confusion between coronary patency and myocardial perfusion. Coronary patency has generally been graded using the Thrombolysis In Myocardial Infarction (TIMI) score, ranging from 0 for total occlusion to 3 for normal "coronary flow" [1]. However, the validity of this angiographic score as the gold standard of thrombolysis success has been challenged. The TIMI study group demonstrated that the TIMI scoring system is far from being objective and reproducible, especially for separation of patients with TIMI 2 and TIMI 3 patency [2]. The authors, using rigorous evaluation of the speed with which coronary arteries fill with dye during angiography (with frame counts), have shown that the TIMI scoring system is poorly reproducible: while the separation of patients with TIMI 2 or 3 flow in the infarct artery from those with TIMI 0-1 flow is fairly reproducible (kappa of 0.84), the interobserver agreement for assessment of TIMI grade 3 flow was only 79%, and it fell to 52% for assessment of TIMI 2 grade flow [2]. Furthermore, the quantitation of TIMI grade flow varies according to the coronary artery considered, and left anterior descending coronary arteries are more likely to be graded as TIMI 2 [2] than right coronary or circumflex arteries. Despite these limitations, angiographic patency is the most widely used technique to assess epicardial "blood flow".

Assessment of Coronary Blood Flow

In the experimental setting, myocardial blood flow can be accurately measured by radioactive microspheres or doppler flow probe. In the clinical setting, measurement of coronary blood flow is often very imprecise, especially during acute myocardial infarction. Coronary blood flow can be accurately assessed by positron emission tomography (PET), but this technique is expensive, not widely accessible, and difficult to use during the acute or early phases of myocardial infarction. Intracoronary doppler flow wires are used to measure basal intra-coronary blood velocity and coronary blood velocity reserve after pharmacological stimulation with adenosine or papaverine. This technique cannot measure absolute blood flow, but is very useful to assess global microvascular reactivity [3]. Acute intra-coronary flow velocity can only be measured in patients undergoing emergency angiography, which limits its use. Magnetic resonance imaging (MRI) is also used to measure myocardial blood flow and detect no-reflow areas [4–7]. Finally, myocardial contrast echocardiography is being investigated as a tool to assess myocardial perfusion during acute phase of myocardial infarction [8, 9]. This technique relies on direct intracoronary injection of contrast agents containing microbubbles, using sonicated radioopaque dyes or specific contrast agents. Simultaneous echocardiography allows opacification of the perfused myocardium through reflection of ultrasonic energy by the air-containing microbubbles located in the myocardial microvasculature. The clinical future of myocardial contrast echocardiography relies upon successful development of intravenously injectable contrast agents able to cross the pulmonary capillary bed, with low ultrasonic attenuation, enabling myocardial opacification of the myocardium [8]. To yield the full potential of these agents, they have to be combined with new emerging ultrasound techniques such as second harmonic imaging, to increase the myocardial contrast enhancement, and intermittent imaging, which limits destruction of the contrast microbubbles by ultrasound. Several experimental and clinical trials of intravenous contrast agents are ongoing using these new techniques, and will hopefully open the way for routine clinical use. A recent experimental study has shown that it was possible to measure absolute myocardial blood flow by continuous infusion of intravenous contrast microbubbles [10].

Assessment of Myocardial Salvage

In the strict sense, the assessment of myocardial salvage requires the measurement of myocardial area at risk (extent of ischemia during coronary artery occlusion) and of final infarct size. These measures are widely used in experimental studies of myocardial ischemia-reperfusion (e.g., with triphenyl tetrazolium chloride, microspheres), but are very difficult to obtain in man, for several reasons. First, the area at risk, by definition, must be measured before coronary artery recanalization. That implies that its measurement must be done immediatly upon patient admission. Second, infarct size is often assessed by either echocardiography or by SPECT, several days after infarction. However, the extent of echocardiographic assynergy, or the size of scintigraphic defect, may overestimate the final infarct, since areas of myocardial stunning and/or hibernation may coexist with areas of myonecrosis. The extent of myocardial salvage in man has been documented for the first time using Technetium Sestamibi scintigraphy [11]. In this study, MIBI-SPECT was performed at admission (assessment of area at risk) and before hospital discharge (final infarct size) in 11 patients receiving and 4 patients not receiving thrombolysis. In patients traeted by thrombolysis, the scintigraphic defect felt from 42±22% at admission to 30±19% at discharge, corresponding to a myocardial salvage of 30%. Conversely, in patients treated with conventional therapy, the scingraphic defect remained unchanged from admission to discharge. These results were confirmed by Behrenbeck et al. [12] in patients with successful (myocardial salvage: 39%) and failed (no salvage) primary PTCA. Despite these interesting results, this method of quantification of myocardial salvage is not easy to use, since it requires injection of a radioactive tracer immediatly upon admission and radionuclide imaging in the intensive care unit. However, myocardial salvage can be approximated by other techniques. For exemple, measurement of MIBI-SPECT or Thallium-SPECT at discharge can be used to compare myocardial salvage in two groups, if one consider than area at risk would have been similar on an acute SPECT. Similarly, myocardial salvage in two groups can be compared using left ventricular ejection fraction, or regional wall motion as assessed by echocardiography.

Coronary Blood Flow as a Predictor of Myocardial Salvage and Improved Prognosis

Coronary Angiographic Patency

The close relationship between coronary angiographic patency and myocardial salvage has been described in the angiographic substudy of the GUSTO trial [13]. The authors showed that the ejection fraction at follow-up was significantly higher (62±14%) in patients with TIMI 3 flow in other patients (55±15%, $P<0.001$). Furthermore, the 30-days mortality was 8.9%, 7.4% and 4.4% in patients with TIMI 0–1, 2, and 3 flow at 90 min, respectively [13]. This finding has been confirmed by many other studies showing a significant lower mortality in patients with TIMI 3 flow, as compared to other patients [14–16]. While patients with incomplete (i.e. TIMI grade 2) and complete (i.e. TIMI 3) patency of the infarct-vessel were initially thought to derive essentially the same benefit from treatment, it has been subsequently demonstrated that benefit is in fact confined to patients with TIMI grade 3 [14, 15, 17]. Anderson et al. reported a meta-analysis of 5 studies on the relation of early coronary patency with outcomes in 3969 patients treated by thrombolysis [18]. The authors confimed that myocardial salvage (as assessed by predischarge left ventricular ejection fraction) was greater in patients with TIMI 3 patency (56%) than in all other patients (52%), even those with epicardial patency but slow flow (TIMI 2). All these studies showed that complete early patency of the infarct vessel is an important goal for reperfusion therapy. However, angiography has serious limitations for judging of the efficacy of reperfusion therapy, however [19]. It only provides a "snapshot" view of coronary patency, even though patency can fluctuate, especially during the early hours of myocardial infarction, with alternating episodes of occlusion and recanalization [20]. More particularly, reocclusion has been shown to happen in 5–15% of patients [21, 22], with negative consequences on left ventricular function and clinical outcome. Furthermore, TIMI 3 flow angiographic recanalization does not always implies myocardial reperfusion. Additional studies using either contrast echocardiography or other techniques such as positron emission tomography, measurement of coronary flow velocity using doppler guidewires, magnetic resonance imaging, or digital angiographic assessment of coronary flow reserve, have corroborated these findings and specifically have confirmed that patients with complete (i.e. TIMI 3) patency form a heterogeneous group of which only a fraction (those patients with the least impairment in microvascular function) displays early recovery of left ventricular function [3, 5, 23–27]. Therefore, myocardial perfusion appears more important than coronary patency [28].

Myocardial Perfusion

The discovery of ischemia/reperfusion-induced microvascular injury challenges the concept of TIMI 3 angiographic patency as the ultimate goal of reperfusion therapy. Reperfusion-induced microvascular injury, jeopardizing myocardial reperfusion, first described on an experimental model by Kloner et al. in 1974 [29] and called the "no-reflow" phenomenon, has been confirmed on other experimental models [30–33]. Using myocardial contrast echocardiography, it has been shown than approximatively 30% of patients with angiographic TIMI 3 flow after angioplasty or thrombolysis during acute myocardial infarction display incomplete myocardial reperfusion [34]. This no-reflow has been shown to be associated with a dramatic decrease in myocardial salvage, and more particularly with a increase in left ventricular volumes and a decrease in ejection fraction [26, 34–36]. Furthermore, no-reflow is a predictor of clinical complications [34]. No-reflow despite epicardial coronary recanalization has been also described by other techniques (MRI, intracoronary doppler, PET) [4, 5].

Enhancement of Coronary Circulation

Coronary Angiographic Patency

The aim of reperfusion therapy is to obtain coronary recanalization as often as possible, and to avoid coronary reocclusion [21, 22].

Choice of Recanalisation Technique

Emergency angioplasty provides higher rate of complete recanalization (TIMI 3 flow) than intravenous thrombolysis, and is associated with improved prognosis [37, 38]. However, using MIBI SPECT, Gibbons et al. only showed a non significant trend towards greater myocardial salvage in patients with anterior myocardial infarction treated by PTCA, as compared to those treated by thrombolysis [11]. This discrepancy between the high rate of coronary patency obtained by primary angioplasty and the absence of significantly higher myocardial salvage may be explained by the small numbers of patients studied (37 patients in the group of patients with anterior infarction). In the group of patients with non anterior myocardial infarctions, the area at risk was possibly too small to observe a consistent myocardial salvage. Finally, there was no systematic predischarge coronary angiography, at the time of the second MIBI-SPECT, to verify the absence of asymptomatic reocclusion. In a study including 142 patients, randomized between thrombolysis and primary PTCA, Zijlstra et al. [39] described a higher predischarge ejection fraction in patients treated by primary PTCA. This difference in terms of left ventricular ejection fraction was not observed in PAMI trial nor in the study of Gibbons et al. [11, 40], but radionuclide angiography was performed 6 weeks after the infarction in these two studies. Finally, it has been shown that myocardial contrast echocardiographic no-reflow was more often observed in patients treated by thrombolysis than by angioplasty [41]. This result confirms that primary PTCA is not only associated with a higher rate of epicardial coronary patency, but also with improved myocardial reperfusion.

Endocoronary Stents

The PAMI Stent Pilot Trial [42] showed that implantation of endocoronary stents was associated with a high rate of TIMI 3 flow (96%) and a decrease in 30 days target-vessel revascularization. Furthermore, Neumann et al. using intracoronary doppler flow wires, showed that patients treated by primary angioplasty + stent presented an important improvement of coronary flow reserve as early as 1 h after recanalization [43]. Finally, Suryapranata et al. [44] recently showed that stenting during primary angioplasty was associated with a significant decrease in target-vessel revascularization (4% vs 17%, $P=0.002$), and in any events (death, reinfarction, target vessel revascularization) at 6 months. Thus, primary stenting is a promising tool to improve epicardial patency and to improve coronary blood flow reserve.

Antiplatelet Therapy

Acute and early reocclusion after coronary angioplasty or intravenous thrombolysis is mostly due to local platelet activation leading to the formation of an obstructive thrombus. Despite the association of heparin and aspirin, early reocclusion is observed in nearly 10% of patients treated successfully by primary angioplasty [21]. New antiplatelets agents are now widely tested as adjunctive therapy during primary angioplasty and thrombolysis. The most widely used antiplatelet agent is abciximab, an inhibitor of platelet glycoprotein IIb/IIIa. A substudy of the EPIC trial, EPIC-MI [45], was the first to show, in a small group of 64 patients, that patients treated by abciximab during and after primary angioplasty had a higher event-free survival than patients receiving placebo. More recently, the larger Rapport trial (483 patients) [46], showed that there was less unplanned stenting and less urgent coronary revascularization in patients treated by abciximab. Furthermore, Neumann et al. [47] showed that patients undergoing primary angioplasty with abciximab had less residual thrombus than placebo patients. They also showed, using intracoronary doppler flow wire, that both basal and peak intracoronary velocity after angioplasty were higher in patients receiving abciximab than in those receiving placebo. Thus, it is highly probable that abciximab, enhancing epicardial patency and coronary flow velocity, could substantially enhance myocardial salvage. Abciximab is also tested as adjunctive therapy to thrombolysis, using lower doses of thrombolytics than in the classical regimens. The preliminary results of TIMI 14 [48] showed that angiographic coronary patency 60 min after thrombolysis was significantly higher in patients receiving abciximab + half-dose (50 mg) of tPA (73%) than in patients receiving the full dose of tPA (100 mg) without abciximab (43%, $P<0.001$). In the same study, the corrected TIMI frame count [2] was higher (indicating slower coronary filling) in patients treated with tPA alone than in patients receiving abciximab (35 vs 28, p 0.03). In the PARADIGM study [49], the authors used another platelet inhibitor, lamifiban, in association with thrombolysis using either streptokinase or tPA, and assessed coronary patency by continuous ECG. They showed that patients receiving lamifiban had a higher rate of 90-minute patency (80%) and a shorter time to steady-state reperfusion (87 min) than patients receiving placebo (63% and 167 min respectively, both <0.05). It appears from these studies than potent antiplatelet therapy as adjunctive therapy to thrombolysis or primary angioplasty allows to address higher rates of stable TIMI 3 flow, and thus an improvement in terms of coronary blood flow. The impact of such treatments on myocardial salvage has to be precised.

Intra-aortic Balloon Pumping

Intra-aortic balloon pumping (IABP) induces an improvement in aortic diastolic pressure [50, 51], and thus may be useful to improve coronary blood flow, which is mainly diastolic [50]. This hypothesis has been confirmed by Kern et al. [51], using intracoronary doppler flow wires in 19 patients (including 11 patients with acute myocardial infarction), who observed increased mean velocity, diastolic velocity, and peak phasic velocity after IABP as compared to before. Some authors have attempted to improve coronary permeability and prevent reocclusion with IABP in patients treated by primary angioplasty. The results of two large studies are discrepant regarding the prevention of reocclusion [52, 53]. Ohman et al. [53] randomized 182 patients with a patent infarct-related artery between 48 h IABP or no balloon. The authors excluded patients with cardiogenic shock or sustained hypotension, which are patients with clinical indications for IABP. They showed that patients with IABP had less reocclusion of the infarct-related artery than patients in the control group (8% vs 21%, $P<0.03$).

Similarly, patients with IABP presented less episodes of recurrent ischemia (4% vs 21%, P=0.001) and needeed less often emergency PTCA (2% vs 11%, P<0.02). However, there was no difference in terms of death, reinfarction or congestive heart failure. In a more recent and larger study [52], Stone et al. randomized 437 high risk patients (age >70 years, three-vessel disease, left ventricular ejection fraction <45%, suboptimal PTCA result) between IABP or no IABP. They excluded patients with preexisting cardiogenic shock. In this study, there was no difference in terms of death, reocclusion, or reinfarction. Similarly, there was no difference in terms of left ventricular ejection fraction at discharge or 6 weeks later. Thus, it appears that IABP may be be reserved to patients with cardiogenic shock or sustained hypotension.

Myocardial Perfusion

Microvascular no-reflow is an anatomical and functional vascular injury, probably induced by abrupt reperfusion rather than by ischemia [30, 54]. Reperfusion injury is probably caused by neutrophils and platelets plugging in myocardial capillaries and oxygen-free-radicals release by activated neutrophils [32, 55–57], which induces endothelial swelling and dysfunction. After reperfusion, blood cells plugging creates a mechanical obstacle to coronary microvascular blood flow [30, 58]. Furthermore, oxygen-free-radicals release may induce a profound endothelium dysfunction [31, 32, 55, 59–61].

Oxygen Free-Radicals Scavengers

Experimental studies in animals have shown that free-radical scavengers, such as superoxide dismutase or catalase, were sometimes associated with an increase in microvascular function and a decrease in infarct size [62–64]. But results of experimental studies are very inconsistent, in part due to methodological variations. In these experimental studies, there was a high disparity in terms of reperfusion delay and length, in SOD dosage, in ischemic models and in species [62]. In man, Flaherty et al. [65] randomized 120 patients treated by primary angioplasty between intracoronary recombinant human superoxide dismutase and placebo administration at the time of recanalization. The authors found no difference in terms of global or regional left ventricular functional recovery at 8 days and 6 weeks. Finally, Forman et al. [61] showed that the oxygen-carrying molecule perfluorochemical (Fluosol) intracoronary administration at the time of recanalization induced a significant decrease in infarct size and a significant improvement in left ventricular functional recovery. However, this study concerned only 12 patients, a population too small to generalize the use of perfluorochemicals in this indication.

Adenosine

Adenosine, which induces microvascular dilatation, is a powerful inhibitor of neutrophil activation, and has been shown to reduce infarct size by improving microvascular perfusion in animal studies. In dogs, Olafsson et al. showed for the first time that infarct size was reduced by almost 70% by intracoronary infusion of adenosine at the time of myocardial reperfusion (infarct size: 9.9% in adenosine group vs 40.9% in control group) [66]. They also observed that myocardial blood flow was significantly higher in dogs receiving adenosine than in control group. Histological study of dog heart showed that adenosine induced an important decrease in neutrophils intravascular accumulation, and that endothelial structure was preserved only in dogs treated by adenosine. These results were entirely confirmed in the same model using intravenous adenosine [67]. Furthermore, in dogs receiving adenosine at the time of reperfusion, coronary blood flow reserve, which reflects the anatomical and/or functional integrity of vascular endothelium, was significantly higher than the coronary flow reserve in control group [68, 69]. More recently, using myocardial contrast echocardiography, Mobarek et al. showed that dogs receiving adenosine at the time of reperfusion were less likely to have echographic no-reflow [70]. Adenosine has also been shown to improve angiographic coronary patency and to reduce scintigraphic infarct size in two clinical studies [71, 72]. Marzilli et al. [71, 73] randomized 40 patients treated by primary angioplasty for acute myocardial infarction between intracoronary adenosine (4 mg in 4 min as soon as balloon deflation) and placebo. They showed that patients treated by adenosine were significantly more likely to have a TIMI 3 flow, and less likely to suffer from congestive heart failure than patients receiving placebo. In a multicentric, randomized, placebo controlled trial, Mahaffey et al. tested the effect of intravenous adenosine in conjonction with thrombolysis, on MIBI-SPECT infarct size and clinical outcomes in 236 patients [72]. The authors showed a non significant decrease in scintigraphic infarct size in patients treated by adenosine (13% vs 19.5%, $P=0.08$). In the subgroup of patients with anterior infarction (77 patients), there was a striking reduction of final infarct size (15% vs 45.5%, $P=0.014$). In a small subset of patients, area at risk has been measured by MIBI-SPECT at admission, allowing the calculation of myocardial salvage. In patients with anterior myocardial infarctions, myocardial salvage was 62% after adenosine, as compared to 15% after placebo ($P=0.015$). Despite this benefit in terms of scintigraphic myocardial salvage, this study failed to show a clinical benefit of adenosine in terms of mortality, congestive heart failure, or recurrence of ischemia. This discrepancy may be related to the relatively low number of patients included.

Other Pharmacological Interventions

In addition, verapamil [74] and nicorandil [75, 76] have been shown to significantly reduce the incidence of no-reflow, as assessed by myocardial contrast echocardiography, and to significantly improve left ventricular functional recovery. Considering the possible role of platelets in microvascular reperfusion injury [57], antiplatelet agents, such as glycoprotein IIb/IIIa receptor antagonists, may also, in addition to contributing to coronary recanalization, impact on myocardial perfusion by decreasing distal microthrombi embolization, inhibiting platelet activation, and decreasing the release of vasoconstricting agents.

Non-pharmacological Interventions

Finally, in addition to pharmacological therapy to reduce no-reflow, there are other perpectives to improve myocardial perfusion in patients with ongoing acute MI, such as therapeutic angiogenesis [77] or preconditioning-like drugs (adenosine may in part act by such a mechanism). The former may preserve a residual myocardial perfusion in the area at risk as a bridge toward delayed coronary recanalisation. The latter may improve the tolerance to ischemia in ischemic myocardium. Preconditioning may also improve endothelial function and myocardial blood flow [54, 78, 79], and thus improve left ventricular functional recovery [80].

In conclusion, restoration of myocardial blood flow at the acute phase of myocardial infarction, as early as possible, is a prerequisite to myocardial salvage. To improve the rate and the quality of epicardial coronary artery recanalization, potent platelet inhibitors and endocoronary stents are now widely used in addition to thrombolysis and primary angioplasty. Despite epicardial coronary recanalization, myocardial reperfusion may be absent. Future direction of clinical pharmacology in the area of myocardial infarction concerns the prevention and the treatment of this no-reflow phenomenon, with promising results obtained with adenosine, nicorandil and verapamil.

References

1. Chesebro J, Knatterud G, Roberts R, et al. (1987) Thrombolysis In Myocardial Infarction (TIMI) trial, Phase I: a comparison between intravenous tissue plasminogen activator and intravenous streptokinase. Circulation 76:142–54
2. Gibson CM, Cannon CP, Daley WL, et al. (1996) TIMI frame count. A quantitative method of assessing coronary artery flow. Circulation 93:879–88
3. Feldman L, Himbert D, Juliard J, et al. (1998) Reperfusion syndrome in acute myocardial infarction: a transient impairment of the microvasculature associated with a larger infarct size and sustained LV dysfunction. J Am Coll Cardiol 31:73 A
4. Nagel E, Underwood R, Pennell D, et al. (1998) New developments in non-invasive cardiac imaging: critical assessment of the clinical role of cardiac magnetic resonance imaging. Eur Heart J 19:1286–93
5. Wu K, Zerhouni E, Judd R, et al. (1998) Prognostic significance of microvascular obstruction by magnetic resonance imaging in patients with acute myocardial infarction. Circulation 97:765–72
6. Wilke N, Simm C, Zhang J, et al. (1993) Contrast-enhanced first pass myocardial perfusion imaging. Correlation between myocardial blood flow in dogs at rest and during hyperemia. Magn Reson Med 29:485–97
7. van der Wall E, van Dijkman P, de Roos A, et al. (1990) Diagnostic significance of gadolinium-DTPA (diethylenetriamine penta-acetic acid) enhanced magnetic resonance imaging in thrombolytic treatment for acute myocardial infarction: its potential in assessing reperfusion. Br Heart J 63:12–7
8. Kaul S (1997) Myocardial contrast echocardiography: 15 years of research and development. Circulation 96:3745–60
9. Karila-Cohen D, Czitrom D, Brochet E, Steg PG (1997) Lessons from myocardial contrast echocardiography studies during primary PTCA. Heart 78:331–2
10. Wei K, Jayaweera AR, Firoozan S, Linka A, Skyba DM, Kaul S (1998) Quantification of myocardial blood flow with ultrasound-induced destruction of microbubbles admistered as a constant venous infusion. Circulation 97:473–83

11. Gibbons RJ, Holmes RR, Reeder GS, et al. (1993) Immediate angioplasty compared with the administration of a thrombolytic agent followed by conservative treatment for myocardial infarction. N Engl J Med 328:685–91
12. Behrenbeck T, Pellikka PA, Huber KC, Bresnahan JF, Gersh BJ, Gibbons RJ (1991) Primary angioplasty in myocardial infarction: assessment of improved myocardial perfusion with technetium-99 m isonitrile. J Am Coll Cardiol 17:365–72
13. The GUSTO Angiographic Investigators (1993) The effect of tissue plasminogen, streptokinase, or both on coronary-artery patency, ventricular function, and survival after acute myocardial infarction. N Engl J Med 329:1615–22
14. Anderson H, Willerson J (1993) Thrombolysis in acute myocardial infarction. N Engl J Med 329:703–9
15. Karila-Cohen D, Juliard JM, Steg PG (1997) Is the "early hazard" related to TIMI 2 patients? Eur Heart J 18 (abstr. suppl):280 (abstract)
16. Karagounis L, Sorensen SG, Menlove RL, Moreno F, Anderson JL, for the TEAM-2 Investigators (1992) Does Thrombolysis In Myocardial Infarction (TIMI) perfusion grade 2 represent a mostly patent or a mostly occluded artery? Enzymatic and electrocardiographic evidence from the TEAM-2 Study. J Am Coll Cardiol 19:1–10
17. Lenderink T, Simoons ML, Van Es GA, et al. (1995) Benefit of thrombolytic therapy is sustained throughout five years and is related to TIMI perfusion grade 3 but not grade 2 flow at discharge. Circulation 92:1110–6
18. Anderson JL, Karagounis LA, Califf RM (1996) Metaanalysis of five reported studies on the relation of early coronary patency grades with mortality and outcomes after acute myocardial infarction. Am J Cardiol 78:1–8
19. Lincoff AM, Topol EJ (1993) Illusion of reperfusion. Does anyone achieve optimal reperfusion during acute myocardial infarction. Circulation 87:1792–805
20. Hackett D, Chierchia S, Maseri A (1987) Intermittent coronary occlusion in acute myocardial infarction: value of combined thrombolytic and vasodilator therapy. N Engl J Med 317:1055–9
21. Garot P, Himbert D, Juliard J, Golmard J, Steg P (1998) Incidence, consequences, and risk factors of early reocclusion after primary and/or rescue percutaneous transluminal coronary angioplasty for acute myocardial infarction. Am J Cardiol 82:554–8
22. Ohman EM, Califf RM, Topol EJ, et al. (1990) Consequences of reocclusion after successful reperfusion therapy in acute myocardial infarction. Circulation 82:781–91
23. Czitrom D, Karila-Cohen D, Brochet E, Faraggi M, Assayag P (1996) Incomplete reperfusion, assessed by myocardial contrast echocardiography, predicts poor wall motion recovery in patients with TIMI 3 patency after primary angioplasty. Circulation 94:I-82 (abstract)
24. Uren N, Crake T, Lefroy D, DeSilva R, Davies G, Maseri A (1994) Reduced coronary vasodilator function in infarcted and normal myocardium after myocardial infarction. N Engl J Med 331:222–7
25. Suryapranata H, Zijlstra F, MacLeod DC, vandenBrand M, deFeyter PJ, Serruys PW (1994) Predictive value of reactive hyperemic response on reperfusion on recovery of regional myocardial function after coronary angioplasty in acute myocardial infarction. Circulation 89:1109–17
26. Ragosta M, Camarano G, Kaul S, Powers ER, Sarembock ER, Gimple LW (1994) Microvascular integrity indicates myocellular viability in patients with recent myocardial infarction. New insights using myocardial contrast echocardiography. Circulation 89:2562–9
27. Kern MJ, Moore JA, Aguirre FV, et al. (1996) Determination of angiographic (TIMI grade) blood flow by intracoronary doppler flow velocity during acute myocardial infarction. Circulation 94:1545–52
28. Steg P, Karila-Cohen D (1998) A paradigm shift for acute myocardial infarction: from coronary patency to myocardial reperfusion. Eur Heart J 19:1282–5
29. Kloner RA, Ganote CE, Jennings RB (1974) The "no-reflow" phenomenon after temporary coronary occlusion in the dog. J Clin Invest 54:1496–508

30. Ambrosio G, Weisman HF, Mannisi JA, Becker LC (1989) Progressive impairment of regional myocardial perfusion after initial restoration of postischemic blood flow. Circulation 80:1846–61
31. Bolli R, Jeroudi MO, Patel BS, et al. (1989) Marked reduction of free radical generation and contractile dysfunction by antioxidant therapy begun at the time of reperfusion. Evidence that myocardial "stunning" is a manifestation of reperfusion injury. Circ Res 65:607–22
32. Bolli R, Triana JF, Jeroudi MO (1990) Prolonged impairment of coronary vasodilation after reversible ischemia. Evidence for microvascular "stunning". Circ Res 67:332–43
33. Jeremy RW, Links JM, Becker LC (1990) Progressive failure of coronary flow during reperfusion of myocardial infarction: documentation of the no reflow phenomenon with positron emission tomography. J Am Coll Cardiol 16:695–704
34. Ito H, Maruyama A, Iwakura K, et al. (1996) Clinical implications of the "no reflow" phenomenon. A predictor of complications and left ventricular remodeling in reperfused anterior wall myocardial infarction. Circulation 93:223–8
35. Brochet E, Czitrom D, Karila-Cohen D, Seknadji P, Faraggi M, Benamer H, Aubry P, Steg PG, Assayag P (1998) Early changes in myocardial perfusion patterns after myocardial infarction: relation with contractile reserve and functional recovery. J Am Coll Cardiol 32: 2011–2017
36. Czitrom D, Karila-Cohen D, Brochet E, Juliard JM, Faraggi M, Assayag P, Aumont MC, Steg PG (1999) Acute assessment of microvascular perfusion patterns by myocardial contrast echocardiography during myocardial infarction: relation to timing and extent of functional recovery. Heart 81:12–16
37. Weaver W, Simes R, Betriu A, et al. (1997) Comparison of primary coronary angioplasty and intravenous thrombolytic therapy for acute myocardial infarction. A quantitative review. JAMA 278:2093–8
38. Michels KB, Yusuf S (1995) Does PTCA in acute myocardial infarction affect mortality and reinfarction rates? A quantitative overview (meta-analysis) of the randomized clinical trials. Circulation 91:476–85
39. Zijlstra F, Jan De Boer M, Hoorntje JCA, Reiffers S, Reiber JHC, Suryapranata H (1993) A comparison of immediate coronary angioplasty with intravenous streptokinase in acute myocardial infarction. N Engl J Med 328:680–4
40. Grines CL, Browne KF, Marco J, et al. (1993) A comparison of immediate angioplasty with thrombolytic therapy for acute myocardial infarction. N Engl J Med 328:673–9
41. Agati L, Voci P, Hickle P, et al. (1998) Tissue-type plasminogen activator versus primary coronary angioplasty: impact on myocardial tissue perfusion and regional function 1 month after uncomplicated myocardial infarction. J Am Coll Cardiol 31:338–43
42. Stone GW, Brodie BR, Griffin JJ, et al. (1998) Prospective, multicenter study of the safety and feasibility of primary stenting in acute myocardial infarction: in-hospital and 30-day results of the PAMI stent pilot trial. Primary Angioplasty in Myocardial Infarction Stent Pilot Trial Investigators. J Am Coll Cardiol 31:23–30
43. Neumann F, Kosa I, Dickfeld T, et al. (1997) Recovery of myocardial perfusion in acute myocardial infarction after successful balloon angioplasty and stent placement in the infarct-related coronary artery. J Am Coll Cardiol 30:1270–6
44. Suryapranata H, van't Hof A, Hoorntje J, de Boer M, Zijlstra F (1998) Randomized comparison of coronary stenting with balloon angioplasty in selected patients with acute myocardial infarction. Circulation 97:2502–5
45. Lefkovits J, Ivanhoe RJ, Califf RM, et al. (1996) Effects of platelet glycoprotein IIb/IIIa receptor blockade by a chimeric monoclonal antibody (abciximab) on acute and six-month outcomes after percutaneous transluminal coronary angioplasty for acute myocardial infarction. EPIC investigators. Am J Cardiol 77:1045–51
46. Brener S, Barr L, Burchenal J, et al. (1998) Randomized, placebo-controlled trial of platelet glycoprotein IIb/IIIa blockade with primary angioplasty for acute myocardial infarction. Circulation 98:734–41

47. Neumann F, Blasani R, Dirschinger J, et al. (1997) Intracoronary stent implantation and antithrombotic regimen in acute myocardial infarction: randomized placebo-controlled trial of the fibrinogen receptor antagonist abciximab. Circulation 96 (supp I):I-398

48. Antman E, Giugliano R, McCabe C, et al. (1998) Abciximab (Reopro) potentiates thrombolysis in ST elevation myocardial infarction: results of TIMI 14 trial. J Am Coll Cardiol 31 (abstract supp):191-A

49. Moliterno D, Harrington R, Krucoff M, et al. (1996) More complete and stable reperfusion with platelet IIb/IIIa antagonism plus thrombolysis for AMI: the PARADIGM trial. Circulation 94 (abstract supp):I-553

50. Gurbel P, Anderson R, MacCord C, et al. (1994) Arterial diastolic pressure augmentation by intra-aortic balloon counterpulsation enhances the onset of coronary artery reperfusion by thrombolytic therapy. Circulation 89:361-5

51. Kern M, Aguirre F, Bach R, Donohue T, Siegel R, Segal J (1993) Augmentation of coronary blood flow by intra-aortic balloon pumping in patients after coronary angioplasty. Circulation 87:500-11

52. Stone GW, Marsalese D, Brodie BR, et al. (1997) A prospective, randomized evaluation of prophylactic intraaortic balloon counterpulsation in high risk patients with acute myocardial infarction treated with primary angioplasty. Second Primary Angioplasty in Myocardial Infarction (PAMI-II) Trial Investigators. J Am Coll Cardiol 29:1459-67

53. Ohman E, George B, White CJ, et al. (1994) Use of aortic counterpulsation to improve sustained coronary artery patency during acute myocardial infarction. Results of a randomized trial. Circulation 90:792-9

54. Richard V, Kaeffer N, Tron C, Thuillez C (1994) Ischemic preconditioning protects against coronary endothelial dysfunction induced by ischemia and reperfusion. Circulation 89:1254-61

55. Kloner RA (1993) Does reperfusion injury exist in humans? J Am Coll Cardiol 21:537-45

56. Braunwald E, Kloner RA (1985) Myocardial reperfusion: a double-edged sword? J Clin Invest 76:1713-9

57. Opie LH (1989) Reperfusion injury and its pharmacologic modification. Circulation 80:1049-62

58. Vanhaecke J, Flameng W, Borgers M, Jang IK, VanderWerf F, DeGeest H (1990) Evidence for decreased coronary flow reserve in viable postischemic myocardium. Circ Res 67:1201-10

59. Forman MB, Puett D, Virmani R (1989) Endothelial and myocardial injury during ischemia and reperfusion: pathogenesis and therapeutic implications. J Am Coll Cardiol 13:450-9

60. Forman MB, Virmani R, Puett DW (1990) Mechanisms and therapy of myocardial reperfusion injury. Circulation 81 (suppl IV):IV 69-IV 78

61. Forman MB, Perry JM, Wilson BH, et al. (1991) Demonstration of myocardial reperfusion injury in humans: results of a pilot study utilizing acute coronary angioplasty with perfluorochemical in anterior myocardial infarction. J Am Coll Cardiol 18:911-8

62. Engler R, Gilpin E (1989) Can superoxide dismutase alter myocardial infarct size. Circulation 79:1137-42

63. Przyklenk K, Kloner R (1989) "Reperfusion injury" by oxygen-derived free radicals? Effect of superoxide dismutase plus catalase, given at the time of reperfusion, on myocardial infarct size, contractile function, coronary microvasculature, and regional myocardial blood flow. Circ Research 64:86-96

64. Ambrosio G, Weisfeldt ML, Jacobus WE, Flaherty JT (1987) Evidence for a reversible oxygen radical-mediated component of reperfusion injury: reduction by recombinant superoxide dismutase administered at the time of reflow. Circulation 75:282-91

65. Flaherty JT, Pitt B, Gruber JW, et al. (1994) Recombinant human superoxide dismutase (h-SOD) fails to improve recovery of ventricular function in patients undergoing coronary angioplasty for acute myocardial infarction. Circulation 89:1982-91

66. Olafsson B, Forman M, Puett D (1987) Reduction of reperfusion injury in the canine preparation by intracoronary adenosine: importance of the nedothelium and the no-reflow phenomenon. Circulation 76:1135-45

67. Pitarys II CJ, Virmani R, Vildibill Jr HD, Jackson EK, Forman MB (1991) Reduction of myocardial reperfusion injury by intravenous adenosine administered during the early reperfusion period. Circulation 83:237–47

68. Babbitt D, Vermani R, Forman M (1989) Intracoronary adenosine administered after reperfusion limits vascular injury after prolonged ischemia in the canine model. Circulation 80:1388–99

69. Norton ED, Jackson EK, Virmani R, Forman MB (1991) Effect of intravenous adenosine on myocardial reperfusion injury in a model with low myocardial collateral blood flow. Am Heart J 122:1283–91

70. Mobarek S, Moreno CA, Revall S, Barbee RW, Murgo JP, Cheirif J (1996) Adenosine reduces micro-vascular damage in the post-reperfusion period: a myocardial contrast echocardiography study. J Am Coll Cardiol 27 (supp A):406 A (abstract)

71. Marzilli M, Gliozheni E, Fedele S, Ungi I, Orsini E, Marraccini P (1997) Beneficial effects of adenosine in acute MI. J Am Coll Cardiol 29 (supp A):133 A (abstract)

72. Mahaffey KW, Puma JA, Barbagelata A, et al. (1999) Adenosine as an adjunct to thrombolytic therapy for acute myocardial infarction. Results of a multicenter, randomized, placebo-controlled trial: the Acute Myocardial Infarction STudy of ADenosine (AMISTAD) Trial. J Am Coll Cardiol 34:711–20

73. Marzilli M, Marraccini P, Gliozheni E, Orsini E, Picano E (1996) Intracoronary adenosine as an adjunct to combined use of primary angioplasty in acute myocardial infarction: beneficial effects on angiographically assessed no-reflow. J Am Coll Cardiol 27 (supp A):81 A (abstract)

74. Taniyama Y, Ito H, Iwakura K, et al. (1997) Beneficial effect of intracoronary verapamil on microvascular and myocardial salvage in patients with acute myocardial infarction. J Am Coll Cardiol 30:1193–9

75. Sakata Y, Kodama K, Komamura K, et al. (1997) Salutary effect of adjunctive intracoronary nicorandil administration on restoration of myocardial blood flow and functional improvement in patients with acute myocardial infarction. Am Heart J 133:616–21

76. Ito H, Taniyama Y, Iwakura K, et al. (1999) Intravenous nicorandil can preserve microvascular integrity and myocardial viability in patients with reperfused anterior wall myocardial infarction. J Am Coll Cardiol 33:654–60.

77. Yanagisawa-Miwa A, Uchida Y, Nakamura F, et al. (1992) Salvage of infarcted myocardium by angiogenic action of basic fibroblast growth factor. Science 257:1401–3

78. DeFily DV, Chilian WM (1993) Preconditioning protects coronary arteriolar endothelium from ischemia-reperfusion injury. Am J Physiol 265:H700-H6

79. Hale S, Kloner R (1992) Effect of ischemic preconditioning on regional myocardial flow in the rabbit heart. Coronary Artery Disease 3:133–40

80. Karila-Cohen D, Czitrom D, Brochet E, Faraggi M, Seknadji P, Himbert D, Juliard JM, Assayag P, Steg PG (1999) Decreased no-reflow in patients with anterior myocardial infarction and pre-infarction angina Eur Heart 20:1724–1730

Subject Index

Printing: Mercedes-Druck, Berlin
Binding: Buchbinderei Lüderitz & Bauer, Berlin